Rawlings, Deirdre.
Fermented foods for
health : use the power
[2013]
33305228581991
bk   11/07/13

WITHDRAWN

FERMENTED FOODS for
HEALTH

Use the Power of Probiotic Foods
to Improve Your Digestion,
Strengthen Your Immunity,
and Prevent Illness

DEIRDRE RAWLINGS, Ph.D., N.D.

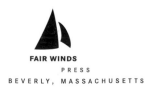

FAIR WINDS
PRESS
BEVERLY, MASSACHUSETTS

© 2013 Fair Winds Press
Text © 2013 Deirdre Rawlings, Ph.D., N.D.
Photography © 2013 Fair Winds Press

First published in the USA in 2013 by
Fair Winds Press, a member of
Quayside Publishing Group
100 Cummings Center
Suite 406-L
Beverly, MA 01915-6101
www.fairwindspress.com

All rights reserved. No part of this book may be reproduced or
utilized, in any form or by any means, electronic or mechanical,
without prior permission in writing from the publisher.

17 16 15 14 13   1 2 3 4 5

ISBN: 978-1-59233-552-7

Digital edition published in 2013
eISBN: 978-1-61058-744-0

Library of Congress Cataloging-in-Publication Data available

Cover design by Kathie Alexander
Book design by Kathie Alexander
Photography by Glenn Scott Photography
Food Styling by Alisa Neely
Preparation of fermented foods by Liz Walkowicz

Printed and bound in China

The information in this book is for educational purposes only.
It is not intended to replace the advice of a physician or medical
practitioner. Please see your health care provider before beginning
any new health program.

CONTENTS

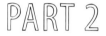

Introduction

As far back as recorded history will take us, we find evidence that humans ate microbiologically fermented foods. Scientists recognized the health benefits associated with fermented foods when Nobel Prize–winning Russian microbiologist Dr. Elie Metchnikoff (1845–1916) credited these foods with boosting immunity and longevity.

Metchnikoff believed that, when consumed, the fermenting *Bacillus* (*Lactobacillus*) positively influenced the microflora of the colon, decreased toxic microbial activities, and improved immunity. He named it *Lactobacillus bulgaricus* after the long-lived, yogurt-loving Bulgarian peasants he studied, and he advocated the wide therapeutic use of these life-giving microorganisms through-out Europe. After Metchnikoff's death in 1916, interest in his work on the fermented food phe-nomena waned as scientists focused on modern therapies such as antibiotics and immunization programs to conquer infectious diseases.

The problem with these modern therapies is that bacteria and viruses are extremely adaptable, and with our efforts to eradicate them, we have pushed them to evolve into stronger adversaries. With the wide use of antibiotics, both in humans and in animals, bacteria has had to undergo rapid mutations in order to evade such strategies, thus making the body more prone to secondary infections. Currently, in the United States alone, 190 million doses of antibiotics are administered each day in hospitals, and more than 133 million

courses of antibiotics are prescribed by doctors to non-hospitalized patients each year. One of the major concerns with the inappropriate or overuse of antibiotics is that they may kill the beneficial bacteria that guard our immune systems, open-ing the door for harmful bacteria to establish themselves in their place. Once this happens, our immune defenses are weakened and our bodies are vulnerable to disease and illness.

Fortunately, there is hope. Consuming probiotic-rich fermented foods is one of the most effec-tive ways we can address these problems and strengthen our immunity against disease to win back our health. When we consume the right nourishment for our bodies' structure, function, and ultimate wellness, good health naturally follows, and fermented foods hold the keys to improved health.

Throughout this book, we'll look at the numerous health benefits from consuming fermented foods and how you can safely use them to proactively address immune disorders, digestive problems, psychiatric disorders, and other chronic condi-tions to positively influence your health and longevity. I've also included a selection of my family's favorite recipes to help start you on your path to wellness.

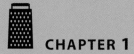

CHAPTER 1

What Is Fermentation?

"Let food be thy medicine, and medicine be thy food."

— HIPPOCRATES

When Hippocrates first made the statement that opens this chapter, he may well have been referring to the medicinal magic of fermented foods. Fermentation isn't a new practice; in fact, it began many centuries ago, making it one of the oldest methods to both preserve and prepare food. Essentially, fermentation facilitated our shift from being solely hunters and gatherers to becoming an agricultural society. The advent of food preservation techniques enabled people to create a future in one place, within a community, because they no longer had to constantly hunt for food.

Fermentation dates back to 5400 BCE with wine-making in Iran, milk fermentation in Babylon circa 5000 BCE, lacto-fermented cabbage in China circa 4000 BCE, leaven (now known as yeast) to raise bread dough in Egypt circa 3000 BCE, and pulque —the oldest alcoholic beverage on the North American continent—in Mexico circa 2000 BCE.

The health benefits from eating fermented foods have been known for centuries. In 76 CE, Roman historian Plinio suggested that fermented milk alleviated gastrointestinal infections. Indeed, Romans obtained the medicinal benefits of lacto-fermented vegetables by eating sauerkraut. Voyagers, from the Roman emperor Tiberius in the first century CE to Captain James Cook in the late eighteen century, relied on sauerkraut to protect their crews from certain intestinal infections and diseases, such as scurvy caused by vitamin C deficiency. Because these voyageurs exported the process around the world, lacto-fermented vegetables include such traditional foods as cabbage in Asia, chutney in India, and relish in America.

The positive health benefits result from the life force inherent in fermented foods: probiotics. Probiotics, which actually means "for life," are living microorganisms that confer a health benefit when consumed in the appropriate amount (more on this later). They manufacture vitamins, especially B complex vitamins such as niacin, biotin, folic acid, and pyridoxine, which support and increase the rate of metabolism; detoxify chemicals; promote cell growth including that of the red blood cells that help prevent anemia; and enhance immune and nervous system function. Probiotics increase the production of enzymes, which improves assimilation and absorption of nutrients from food, particularly proteins and fats. They are especially effective in crowding out growth of pathogenic microorganisms, thereby boosting immune system response.

Fermentation Spans the Globe

The art of fermentation has been core to civilizations across the world for millennia. Traditional fermented foods have formed a stable component of these diverse diets. Worldwide, people enjoy beers and wines, breads, cheeses, and vinegars—all the products of fermentation. But many cultures have a distinctive fermented food that's a fundamental part of their diets: sauerkraut in Central Europe, kimchi in Korea, miso in Japan, olives and cured meats in the Mediterranean countries, yogurt and chutney in India, pickled herring in Scandinavia, Vegemite in Australia, tarama (fermented roe) in the Far Eastern countries, and let's not overlook pickles and sourdough bread in the United States.

THE PROCESS OF FERMENTATION

Fermentation happens when microorganisms (natural bacteria and some yeasts) feed on the sugar and starch in food, converting them into lactic acid in a process known as lacto-fermentation. There are several types of fermentation (which I'll briefly discuss on page 7), but lacto-fermentation provides the most health benefits and, therefore, is the type we will focus on in this book.

From a biochemical perspective, fermentation involves the metabolic breakdown of a nutrient anaerobically (without the use of oxygen). This breakdown produces ethanol, acids, gases, and other precursor molecules, which act as intermediate compounds in a chain of enzymatic reactions, from which a more stable or definitive product is formed. In a broader sense, lacto-fermentation creates beneficial bacteria, enzymes, vitamins, and various strains of probiotics (live beneficial microorganisms). An added benefit just happens to be an increased shelf life of food. Interestingly, fermentation doesn't just encompass one basic process—it's nearly as diverse as the range of foods it produces.

Fermented Food Classifications

Not only does fermentation contribute to a diverse diet, but it also preserves, enriches, and detoxifies foods. It is the life force—that is, live bacteria, yeasts, and molds—behind fermented foods that confers its beneficial impact on your health. The sheer number and variety of these microorganisms is what creates the great diversity of fermented foods, which can generally be broken down into seven categories:

1. **Cultured vegetable protein.** These usually consist of legumes, such as soybeans, which are used to produce tempeh, an Indonesian staple dating back two thousand years. Tempeh is made from cooked, hulled, fermented soybeans bound together with a mold that makes soy easier to digest. The result is a pressed cake, often used as a meat substitute, that can be sliced, grated, chopped, or even slipped onto a skewer for the grill.

2. **High-salt-content, meat-flavored fermentation pastes.** These usually consist of salty and savory meat-flavored, protein-bound grains and legumes, such as soybeans, that are soaked, mashed, cooked, and left to ferment to make pastes and sauces. Most of these fermentations originated in Asian countries. Examples include soy sauce, miso, shoyu, Vietnamese mam, Indonesian trassi, and Malaysian belachan.

3. **Alcohol fermentations.** These appear in biblical references as fermented wine. In this naturally occurring biological process, sugars, such as glucose, fructose, and sucrose, are converted into cellular energy by yeasts when placed in an environment absent of oxygen, whereby the microorganisms also produce ethanol (alcohol) and carbon dioxide as their metabolic waste products. We derive wine by fermenting the natural sugars found in grapes. Rum is produced by fermenting sugarcane, and whiskey, vodka, and beers are all produced by fermenting grain.

4. **Vinegar fermentation.** This type of fermentation process results when you expose alcohol (ethanol) to oxygen. Vinegar is produced by a group of bacteria known as *Acetobacter*, which convert the alcohol into acetic acid, or vinegar. You may have experienced this type of fermentation if you've ever left a bottle of wine open for too long! Examples of acetic acid fermentation include apple cider vinegar, wine vinegars, coconut water vinegar, and African palm vinegar.

Food Preservation

Fermentation preserves food in a much more beneficial manner than the more commonly relied upon food sterilization technique, pasteurization. While pasteurization detracts from a food's nutritional value—mainly by killing off enzymes, as well as friendly and useful germs alike—fermentation actually increases it (more on this later in the chapter). As a bonus, fermenting your own foods enables you to purchase local raw foods and store them for future use without worrying about them spoiling.

5. **Alkaline-fermented foods.** These are less common foods made from various raw ingredients that are predominantly consumed in Southeast Asia and African countries. One such example is Japanese natto, made from cooked soybeans, or ugba from African oil beans. The proteins in the raw materials are broken down into their component amino acid and peptide parts, releasing ammonia and increasing the pH of the product, which results in the strong smell associated with these fermentations.

6. **Leavened breads.** These are made from fermented grains, such as wheat or rye, which employ naturally occurring yeasts and *Lactobacilli* to raise the dough and create sourdough. Because the *Lactobacilli* produce lactic acid, sourdoughs produce a mildly sour taste, unlike breads made with baker's yeast. The fermented mix of grain and water, called a "sourdough starter," can be saved and used to start another batch of dough. The history of making leavened breads dates back to ancient times, with records as far back as six thousand years ago.

7. **Lactic acid fermentation.** Lactic acid fermentation occurs when bacteria convert sugars present in the food into cellular energy and lactate, or lactic acid. Lactic acid is a natural preservative that inhibits putrefying bacteria, and the process is one of the most significant forms of fermentation in the food industry. Examples of vegetable lactic acid fermentations include sauerkraut, cucumber pickles, olives, kimchi, kefir, yogurt, soymilk, buttermilk, cheeses, and tofu.

We have been harnessing this natural process to ferment traditional foods for thousands of years. The Greeks deemed this ancient process "alchemy," to capture the magical transformations that occurred during fermentation. The earliest form of lactic acid fermentation is believed to have been milk fermented into yogurt, kefir, cheeses, and buttermilk. Raw milk, which is unpasteurized, sours quite rapidly due to the natural fermentation conducted by lactic acid bacteria. The bacteria convert lactose (milk sugar) into lactic acid, which serves as a preservative. Lactic acid is a natural antibiotic that keeps spoiling organisms away from the naturally preserved foods that contain it.

Yet the benefits of lacto-fermentation do not stop at preservation. Lacto-fermentation creates an incredible array of flavors and textures. *Lactobacilli*—the most important lactic acid–producing bacteria—proliferate during the process of fermentation, making fermented foods so healthful. Because *Lactobacilli* increase the digestibility of vegetables by providing their own natural enzymes, our bodies do not have to completely rely on the digestive system to metabolize foods. These bacteria also increase the natural vitamin content of vegetables and produce antibiotics and cancer-fighting agents. Lactic acid also facilitates the proliferation of healthy gastrointestinal tract flora that are so integral to our well-being. We'll be looking at each of these amazing abilities throughout part 1.

BACTERIA IN THE BODY

Bacteria don't reside only in food. A whole category of living things, called microorganisms, inhabit the human body. Everything from our digestive systems to our skin is home to millions of these microorganisms. Many of these microorganisms are essential for our health and live in equilibrium within our bodies in a relationship that has evolved over billions of years. There are more than 10 trillion cells in the human body, but approximately ten times that number of bacterial cells. On the whole, the microbes we host are known as our microflora.

Some of these organisms perform tasks that are useful for the human host, such as preventing growth of harmful species, regulating the development of the gut, producing important vitamins, and strengthening the immune system. A few species of bacteria, however, are pathogenic and cause infectious diseases; for example, *Salmonella typhi* causes typhoid, *Varicella zoster* causes chicken pox, and *Mycobacterium tuberculosis* causes tuberculosis. But the majority of bacteria species have no known beneficial or harmful effect.

After birth the normal bacterial flora in humans usually develops, leading to the stable populations of bacteria that make up normal adult flora. The composition of the normal flora in any part of the body is determined mainly by the nature of the local environment, by its pH, temperature, oxygen, water, and nutrient levels. In a healthy individual, only the internal tissues—blood, brain, muscle—are normally free of microorganisms. The surface tissues—skin and mucous membranes—however, are constantly in contact with environmental organisms and can become readily colonized by various bacteria.

Your body is therefore a complicated ecosystem featuring a symbiotic relationship with these bacteria and their genes; "microbiome" refers to both the bacteria and their genes. We, as hosts, provide the environment to sustain these bacteria, and we rely on them to fulfill pivotal processes we could not survive without. For example, the microbiome possesses compounds that we need but would not otherwise be able to produce, such as vitamins and anti-inflammatories, useful for preventing growth of harmful species, regulating the development of the gut, producing important vitamins, and strengthening the immune system.

We are constantly exposed to microorganisms that are on the lookout for a host body that can help sustain and increase their population. Their mode of entry can be through air, water, food, and person-to-person contact. This constant exposure to new microorganisms makes it necessary to have a strong defense to actively prevent colonization of the disease-causing microorganisms. Because they are rich in beneficial microorganisms, fermented foods can bolster that defense.

Development of the Body's Normal Microflora

Your skin and mucous membrane—the linings of all body passages and cavities that are exposed to the external environment and internal organs—contain a large amount of microflora that are considered the human body's natural microflora. During birth, humans first become colonized by normal microflora. Within the uterus, the baby is kept sterile until the mother's water breaks, and as the birth process begins, so, too, does the colonization of the microflora on the body's surfaces. The microorganisms present in the mother's vagina pass on to the baby, and the colonization of these beneficial microorganisms take up any available space and all nutrition, thereby limiting the colonization of potentially pathogenic microorganisms. During Cesarean deliveries, this transfer is completely absent. These babies commonly acquire and are colonized with flora from the hospital's environment and, therefore, their flora may differ from their mothers'. Either way, feeding and handling of the newborn, as well as ordinary contact with bedding and even family pets, begins the establishment of the stable normal flora on the surfaces of the baby's skin, mouth, and intestines. Breastfeeding is essential for populating the baby's gut with balanced, healthy flora; breast milk contains *Bifidobacterium bifidum*, which produces lactic acid and protects the infant against both intestinal and respiratory diseases. As the baby's intestinal microflora flourishes, it contributes to the development and function of the gut's mucosal barrier, which builds resistance against colonization from various disease-causing microorganisms.

For Optimum Health and Survival

Fermented foods are abundant in essential vitamins, minerals, enzymes, and antioxidants that are all enhanced through the process of fermentation. Studies show that the nutrients in fermented foods may even play a role in mitigating the risk of certain cancers, particularly those of the stomach and intestines. There's further evidence that fermented foods reduce overall inflammation in the body. Inflammation is the body's first response to cell injury, body pain, invading pathogens, or some other stressor, in a protective attempt to remove the injurious stimuli and initiate a healing response. Too much inflammation in the body is mostly the result of an overactive immune system that's running out of control. Left unchecked, it can result in common conditions like allergies, autoimmune disease, lupus, and rheumatoid arthritis. I'll explain this more in depth in the coming chapters.

An Overview of Intestinal Flora

The most extensive population of microbes in the body exists in the gastrointestinal tract, where approximately 80 percent of our microflora live. Average adults possess 2½ to 3 pounds (1.1 to 1.4 kg) of bacteria in the gut, which collectively perform innumerable digestive functions that we could not perform on our own, such as:

- improving the bioavailability of nutrients from food

- strengthening immunity

- manufacturing B-complex vitamins

- aiding absorption of vitamins and minerals

- protecting the integrity of the intestinal lining

- producing antiviral substances

- producing antifungal substances

- neutralizing endotoxins (compounds found in the cell walls of bacteria that protect them from threat and are released when the bacteria die; many of these toxins cause health problems)

- regulating cytokines (chemical messengers that help regulate the nature and intensity of the immune system's response) so as to reduce inflammation in the body

- neutralizing potentially carcinogenic nitrites in the digestive tract

- extracting calcium from dairy products

The microflora in the gut are divided into four main groups. The first two are the essential, or beneficial, flora, which are in large number in healthy individuals. These two groups are predominantly made up of *Bifidobacteria* and *Lactobacilli*, and together the presence of these two bacteria is considered to be one of the most important aspects of a healthy intestinal microflora. The third group of microflora is those we ingest through food or drink, and the fourth group, yeasts and molds, are not bacteria but rather fungi.

Bifidobacteria

Bifidobacteria are normal inhabitants of the human colon and vaginal area. There are around thirty different species identified within this group, the most commonly known in the body being *B. bifidum*, *B. breve*, *B. longum*, and *B. infantis*. These friendly microbes are about seven times more numerous than *Lactobacilli* in a healthy adult gut but are found in especially large numbers in the intestines of breastfed babies who receive *Bifidobacteria* through their mother's milk. (In bottle-fed babies, *Bifidobacteria* are not as predominant.) These good microorganisms prevent the colonization of highly virulent strains of microorganisms that could lead to infection, particularly in the stomach. Studies show that *Bifidobacteria* exhibit strong immune-modulating effects, suggesting that they are strong boosters of immune system function. Foods that contain *Bifidobacteria* include fermented dairy products such as yogurt and kefir, fermented vegetables such as sauerkraut, and beverages such as kombucha.

Lactobacilli

Lactobacilli is a large family of important bacteria that produce lactic acid. These are found mainly in the small intestine, mucous membranes of the mouth, throat, nose, and upper respiratory tract, vagina, and genital area. The most commonly known members of the *Lactobacilli* family are *L. acidophilus*, *L. bulgaricus*, *L. rhamnosus*, *L. plantarum*, *L. reuteri*, *L. johnsonii*, *L. delbrueckii*, *L. salivarius*, and *L. casei*. *Lactobacillus acidophilus* are the main residents of the small bowel, where they are engaged in the cell renewal process to keep the gut walls healthy and intact, and they're usually present in large colonies in pregnant women. These bacteria are also present in the vagina and are responsible for its low pH, an acidic environment that inhibits the growth of pathogenic microorganisms.

Apart from lactic acid, *Lactobacilli* produce many active substances in the gut, such as lactase and hydrogen peroxide—a naturally powerful antiseptic, antiviral, antifungal, and antibacterial agent that prevents pathogens from taking hold in the gut. Studies show that *Lactobacilli* are strong triggers of anti-inflammatory cytokine production. Cytokines are proteins produced by white blood cells, namely macrophages and monocytes, which are key players in the immune response to foreign invaders such as bacterial infections. They are found in fermented foods such as yogurt, raw milk, fermented meat, vegetables, fruits, sourdough bread, and beverages such as kombucha.

Ingestible Microflora

The third group of microflora, those we acquire through food and drink, may be quite large and include several species of bacteria that can cause a wide variety of infections in both humans and animals through either toxin production or invasion. These bacteria are not generally associated with fermented foods (which negate their toxic effects), but rather with contaminated or improperly stored foods. They are a common cause of food poisoning in people whose gut microflora is imbalanced or contains insufficient numbers of the friendly bacteria. The composition of this group varies from person to person, though it is generally made up of the following:

- *Bacteroides*
- *Peptococci*
- *Staphylococci*
- *Streptococci*
- *Bacilli*
- *Clostridia*
- *Enterobacteria*
- *Fuzobacteria*
- *Eubacteria*
- *Catenobacteria*
- Yeasts

In healthy people, these incoming bacteria usually pass through the gastrointestinal tract. However, if poor health has compromised the composition or number of beneficial flora that regulate these microbes, then this group could grow quite large and adversely affect health. For example, some *Streptococci* species are normally associated with mild illnesses such as strep throat; however, if good gut flora is weak, it may allow the *Streptococci* to stay for too long or multiply in the small intestine. In rare cases, a more severe illness can occur, such as streptococcal toxic shock syndrome, which causes rapid blood pressure drop and organ failure.

Fungal Microflora

The human body is also host to yeast, single-cell fungi related to molds, which is naturally occurring and not specifically dangerous in balanced amounts. (Beneficial yeasts, you'll recall, are also responsible for fermenting many different foods, such as sourdough bread, wine, and beer.) Yeasts are typically larger than most bacteria and are found throughout nature, anywhere from the air to the soil. While some yeasts, such as *Candida albicans*, can have detrimental health effects, others, such as *Saccharomyces* and certain *Aspergillus*, facilitate healthful food fermentations through the production of enzymes.

● Yeast Enters the Medical Annals

In 1923, French microbiologist Henri Boulard observed a group of Indo–Chinese treating choleric diarrhea with a tea made from lychee and mangosteen. What he discovered was a new strain of yeast, Saccharomyces boulardii. *He returned home and patented it as a probiotic antidiarrheal drug, which is still used today.*

Molds are a type of fungi that live on plants and foods, which, when eaten, can take up residence in humans. The *Penicillium* genus of mold is the most well known because some species contain the active ingredient penicillin, which is attributed to its strong antibacterial properties. Just as with bacteria and yeasts, molds are also well known for spoiling food and emitting undesirable toxins, and the *Aspergillus* species of mold are often the culprits of these undesirable effects. Beneficial molds add flavor to foods, such as certain cheeses, and produce enzymes, such as amylase, that can be used to make bread.

THE FUTURE IS FERMENTED FOODS

Although our bodies contain more than 100 trillion bacteria, from more than 400 different species, we still have much to discover about them. Comprehensive sequencing studies, including the National Institute of Health's ongoing Human Microbiome Project, are essential to extending our knowledge of these microorganisms. However, what we know with certainty is these living bacteria require a specific environment to flourish, and diet has a direct impact on gastrointestinal system health. Although much has yet to be learned about the interplay between disease and microorganisms, the evidence suggests there is a clear link between the two. In the next chapter, we'll learn about the gastrointestinal and immune systems, how they intertwine, and how fermented foods can benefit them both.

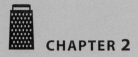

CHAPTER 2

Your Immune and Digestive Systems: Your Internal Ecosystem at Work

"Natural forces within us are the true healers of disease."

— HIPPOCRATES

In the last chapter, we covered fermentation—what it is and how it acts on food. We talked about bacteria—how bacterial cells outnumber human cells in our bodies and how not all bacteria are bad. Then we looked further at the normal microflora that reside in our guts. Now we're going to focus on the two main body systems that keep us well: the immune system and the gastrointestinal system.

You might be somewhat familiar with the inner workings of the immune system, from the macrophages to the lymphocytes. Or you may just know that it's what keeps you from falling ill and helps you get better when you do get sick. But you may surprised to learn the bulk of the immune system resides in the gastrointestinal tract, and our guts are actually our number one defense when it comes to preventing illness. Our guts and our immune systems work in tandem to keep us well, and they do this by trafficking in beneficial bacteria.

YOUR BODY AS A SOCIAL NETWORK

The human immune system defends the body and protects against disease-causing organisms. It is a complex network made up of specialized cells, proteins, tissues, and organs located throughout the body, from your eyes and skin to your nasal passages and lymphatic fluids. About 75 to 80 percent of the immune system is housed in the gastrointestinal tract. White blood cells called lymphocytes are important members of the immune system. They are located throughout the body and in a healthy person are found in abundance in the digestive wall. Lymphocytes are responsible for identifying, attacking, and killing dangerous microbes.

But let's not downplay the immune system's second role: in addition to defending against invaders, it protects the body from invaders ever taking root. The beneficial bacteria in the gut produce gases and various acids that benefit the intestine and other body systems and reduce the pH of the colon, making the environment less suitable for pathogenic bacteria. The beneficial bacteria can also engage lymphocytes (both T and B cells) into action to kill potential invaders and support immune system defense. *Lactobacilli* have been specifically shown to excite immunoreactive macrophages (a type of white blood cell that "eats" foreign material and invaders in the body) into action, thereby boosting immune system function. A person with damaged gut flora has far fewer lymphocytes in the gut wall, which leaves not only the gut but also the whole body poorly protected.

An important role of lymphocytes in the gut wall is to produce antibodies, also known as immunoglobulins, used by the immune system to identify and neutralize foreign particles such as bacteria and viruses. The most important antibody in the gut is secretory immunoglobulin A (sIgA). IgA is produced in mucosal linings (breathing passages, nose, throat), secretions (saliva, tears, sweat), the genitourinary tract (bladder, urethra, vagina), colostrum in breast milk, and of course, mucous membranes that line the gut wall, than all other types of antibodies combined. It is also found in small amounts in blood. Its job is to protect mucous membranes from invading pathogens by destroying and inactivating them.

The dominance of IgA production in the gastrointestinal mucosa depends on colonization with beneficial microflora. As the level of beneficial bacteria compared to pathogenic bacteria increases, the level of proinflammatory cytokines (immune-modulating agents) and production of IgA decreases. In fact, any attempt to replace or supplement the body's damaged microflora reduces the effects of disease-causing microbes. Fermented foods contain the essential beneficial microorganisms required to ward off disease and fight everyday threats to our health. An abundant supply of these microorganisms builds a strong, resilient immune system and helps us bounce back quickly from the inevitable occasional illness. Daily consumption of lacto-fermented–rich foods, such as yogurt, sauerkraut, kefir, and kimchi, containing *L. acidophilus* and *Bifidobacteria*, supports the abundant production of a healthy army of defending antibodies.

Neonatal Probiotics

Fermented foods and probiotics are particularly effective during pregnancy and breastfeeding. Pregnant women often suffer from a range of discomforts due to digestive issues, which can easily be relieved by introducing probiotic foods into the diet. Probiotic-enriched foods further stimulate the production of immunoglobulin A, a crucial component of the immune system that helps defend against allergens and aids in proper functioning of the baby's digestive system. Breastfeeding is fundamental to establishing an infant's health, partially because it helps create the composition of healthy gut bacteria.

THE ROAD TO HEALTH IS PAVED WITH GOOD DIGESTION

The digestive system is the center of your internal ecosystem. With a surface area that is about the size of a tennis court, a properly functioning gut is the foundation of good health. The digestive system's function is to process essential nutrients—such as proteins, essential fatty acids, vitamins, minerals, and enzymes—from the foods you eat into particles that your cells can use for energy, growth, repair, and maintenance. This breakdown of nutrients occurs when specific digestive enzymes, produced naturally by our bodies, are mixed with the food. Enzymes are catalysts that speed the breakdown of nutrients from foods to supply energy to cells. These construction workers use the nutrients as building materials to construct your body. Simply put, enzymes run everything that goes on inside of you to sustain life. We'll discuss these important workers and their amazing restorative and regenerative healing powers in more detail in chapter 3.

Although the old saying "You are what you eat" is primarily true, what truly matters is what you absorb and assimilate from what you eat. If you don't absorb nutrients well, all other health factors and body systems are undermined. The health of your cells is determined by the continued nourishment they receive from the foods you eat, so your number one priority is to eat nutritious foods that your digestive system can easily break down and absorb.

Fermented foods, then, are of utmost value because they furnish a rich supply of beneficial microflora and enzymes that combine to support the digestive process. Their beneficial microorganisms inhibit the growth of pathogenic bacteria by secreting large amounts of lactic acid, making the environment too acidic and unsuitable for pathogens. The lactic acid–producing bacteria, along with the help of enzymes in fermented foods, manufacture essential vitamins in your body: B1, B2, B3, B5, B6, B12, A, and K, all of which play important roles in strengthening immune system function and promoting healthy metabolism.

Again, the digestive tract is home to some 100 trillion living bacteria of more than 400 different species, each of which has many types of strains. Approximately 20 types make up three-quarters of the total. Because these microorganisms are living, they require a certain environment in order to thrive. A large percentage are anaerobic, meaning they do not need oxygen to survive (making the gut a good place to set up house-keeping). Some are aerobic, meaning they require oxygen to survive. A third group produces lactic acid and can be either anaerobic or aerobic. Again, it is the lactic acid–producing bacteria that help acidify the intestinal tract and protect us from overgrowth of harmful bacteria.

Most of the human digestive tract, including the intestines, colon, pancreas, and saliva, is in its proper and healthy balance when there is a preponderance of healthy microorganisms, including predominantly *Lactobacillus* and *Bifidobacteria*. Raw lacto-fermented vegetables, such as cabbage, beets, carrots, garlic, cauliflower, and garlic, all contain beneficial microorganisms that support your digestive system. By preventing colonization of pathogenic bacteria and yeasts, these microorganisms protect the integrity of the intestinal lining by preventing toxins from seeping through the cell walls of the intestines and poisoning organs and tissues throughout the body. When the organs become poisoned, their ability to assimilate nutrients and function properly is diminished. Maintaining integrity of intestinal walls helps regulate peristalsis and bowel movements, ensuring toxins are eliminated regularly through the proper channels.

Leaky Gut

Modern diets, with their high concentrations of processed foods and preservatives, wreak havoc on the gut walls by damaging the villi—finger-like protrusions in the intestine that help absorb nutrients from food more efficiently. The result is inflammation, which leads to dysbiosis, or an upset and imbalance in the normal microflora that allows harmful bacteria and yeast to multiply uncontrollably. The presence of dysbiosis leads to increased intestinal permeability, or what is more commonly referred to as "leaky gut syndrome." In other words, when the microflora become imbalanced, the walls or lining of the digestive tract become damaged, and because the intestinal membrane is so thin, food substances or larger molecules can pass through the walls directly into the bloodstream, bypassing normal digestive processes. This can lead to malabsorption of the important nutrients your body needs to sustain itself.

Additionally, a leaky gut raises alarm signals to the natural killer cells in your immune system, which then tag such food substances or molecules as foreign and trigger an antibody reaction. This sets up food intolerance and sensitivity reactions whenever you eat those same foods in the future. A leaky gut can also allow disease-causing bacteria to invade and colonize in other parts of the body, causing all sorts of autoimmune-related problems and contributing to a variety of symptoms and disorders, such as inflammatory bowel disorder, food allergies, Crohn's disease, malnutrition, lupus, and inflammatory joint disease or arthritis.

Conditions Tied to Leaky Gut

Leaky gut syndrome is receiving increasing attention as the hard-to-deal-with factor in patients being treated for food intolerances. Hyper-permeability is associated with gastrointestinal tract disorders such as Crohn's disease, celiac disease, irritable bowel syndrome (IBS), gluten intolerance, lactose intolerance, yeast infections, chronic constipation or gas, and chronic giardiasis (a chronic intestinal infection caused by the water-borne parasite Giardia lamblia). A growing body of evidence shows that all of these conditions can be helped through the addition of good bacteria—and the way to get them is by adding fermented foods to the daily diet.

OUR SILENT PARTNERS FOR GOOD HEALTH

Our digestive tract is vulnerable to infection because it is open at both ends and plays host to anything we ingest, as well as anything else entering from our external environment. We can thank our friendly bacteria—our microflora—for coating the entire tract, thereby creating a physical barrier against unwanted microbes and viruses. Additionally, the wall of the gut maintains a pH from 4.0 to 5.0. This acidic environment is not conducive to the growth of pathogenic materials that require a more basic environment to thrive. This group of friendly microflora also neutralizes toxins derived from pathogenic microbes in our ingested foods. But their protection of our digestive tract doesn't stop there. Microflora also produce specific substances designed to break down each type of intruder that threatens our immune system. In doing so, they alert our immune system to get ready for battle.

The normal gut microflora provides a major source of energy and nourishment for the cells lining the digestive tract—and ultimately, the rest of your body. Apart from keeping the gut wall in good shape, the healthy microflora populating this wall take an active role in the digestion and absorption of foods. In addition to this, they are able to manufacture essential vitamins, all of which produce immune-strengthening substances. Without the good microbes, food is not properly absorbed and essential nutrients cannot be assimilated, which leads to malnourishment. When this happens, your body's defense systems are quickly lowered as cells are starved of energy and are further denied growth, repair, and maintenance. Fatigue and sickness quickly ensue, which provides the opportunistic flora that live in the gut, under tight control by the beneficial flora, favorable conditions that permit them to gain the upper hand. The entire immune system then gets out of balance and is therefore weakened, which makes the person immune compromised.

You can see, from the previous example, just how important balanced microflora are to your well-being. This normal microflora and the human body have a dynamic, mutually beneficial relationship. The microorganisms gain shelter, nutrition, and transport, and they flourish in the stable environment of the living host. In turn, the microorganisms help your body by aiding in digestion, stimulating your immune system, and protecting your body's tissues from colonization by harmful microbes. The presence of these microorganisms elicits an immune response that keeps the body's defense mechanism active so that when a disease-causing microorganism—called an antigen, which can be bacteria, fungi, viruses, or parasites—infects the body, your immune response will be faster and of greater intensity.

When There's a Lack of Friendly Microbes

So what happens when you are deficient in friendly bacteria? To start, you would be unable to digest fiber, and as a result you would become deficient in certain vitamins. Such deficiencies bring a whole host of conditions such as anemia, a condition in which a person has insufficient red blood cells to carry oxygen to the body's tissues. There are several mechanisms behind this. First, there's an overgrowth of pathogenic bacteria (most commonly *Escherichia coli*, and *Streptococcus* and *Enterococcus* species) that thrive on iron before your body can utilize or absorb it. Second, with a decreased amount of the friendly microflora and overgrowth of the pathogenic bacteria in your gut, your body cannot break down fiber, which can cause malabsorption problems. It may also induce a high frequency of diarrhea, which can upset the body's electrolyte balance and ability to utilize important minerals and vitamins. In addition to the resulting deficiency in blood-supporting vitamins and minerals, new bacteria will move in that thrive on iron, and trying to supplement your diet with iron will only fortify these pathogenic bacteria.

Here are other nutrients and vitamins that can become deficient from a lack of microflora to digest fiber:

- magnesium (involved in several hundred enzymatic reactions, many of which contribute to production of energy and cardiovascular function)
- zinc (needed for the body's immune system to function properly)
- selenium (protects the immune system by preventing the formation of free radicals)
- copper (aids in the formation of bone, hemoglobin, and red blood cells)
- calcium (vital for the formation of strong bones and teeth and for the maintenance of healthy gums)
- manganese (needed for protein and fat metabolism, a healthy immune system, and blood sugar regulation)
- sulfur (disinfects the blood, helps the body resist pathogenic bacteria, and protects cells)
- phosphorus (needed for blood clotting, bone and tooth formation, cell growth, normal heart rhythm, and kidney function)
- potassium (important for a healthy nervous system, a regular heart rhythm, and stable blood pressure)
- sodium (necessary for maintaining proper blood pH and for stomach, nerve, and muscle function)
- vitamin B1 (thiamine) (needed in the production of hydrochloric acid, which is important for proper digestion)

- vitamin B2 (riboflavin) (necessary for red blood cell formation, antibody production, cell respiration, and growth)

- vitamin B3 (niacin) (aids in the production of hydrochloric acid for the digestive system)

- vitamin B6 (pyridoxine) (involved in more bodily functions, both physically and mentally, than almost any other single nutrient)

- vitamin B12 (important for alleviating fatigue, stress, and anxiety)

- vitamin C (required for at least three hundred metabolic functions in the body; more on this antioxidant in chapter 3)

- vitamin A (enhances immunity)

- vitamin D (necessary for growth)

- folic acid (important for alleviating fatigue, stress, and anxiety, and has disease-prevention properties)

- omega-3 fatty acids, including alpha-linolenic and eicosapentaenoic acid (EPA) (essential in the transmission of nerve impulses and needed for the normal development and functioning of the brain)

- omega-6 fatty acids, which include linoleic and gamma-linolenic acids (play an important role in brain function, skin and hair growth, bone health, reproduction, and healthy metabolism)

- omega-9 fatty acids (play an important role in the production of prostaglandins, lowers LDL cholesterol levels, and used to build omega-3s and -6s in the body)

- taurine (a building block of all the other amino acids that make up protein. It is needed for the digestion of fats, the absorption of fat-soluble vitamins, and the control of serum cholesterol levels.)

Fermented foods introduce beneficial microorganisms and other healing substances such as vitamins, minerals, and enzymes into the body; all of these restore the balance of the intestinal flora and improve digestive health. Increasing evidence suggests that the gastrointestinal tract and digestive system play an integral role in our health. Because the friendly bacteria left behind as a by-product of fermentation reside mainly in the gut, they can support digestion and absorption of nutrients. The community of beneficial microorganisms within the body is what helps manufacture essential vitamins and minerals and provide important enzymes necessary for digestion. And when gastrointestinal health is promoted, overall health is supported.

MORE THAN A BELLYACHE

Unfortunately, the highly processed Western diet that many of us grew up on is mostly devoid of naturally occurring nutrients such as essential fatty acids, minerals, vitamins, enzymes, fiber, and antioxidants. The growth of our industrialized-food consumption during the past century is partly to blame, as is the increase in usage of anti-biotic drugs that change the makeup of our gut flora. The health of your digestive system and its intestinal microflora is what determines whether you receive maximum nourishment from the foods you eat, which in turn affects the immune system and your entire body. A faulty digestive system is behind most, if not all, of these diseases:

- heartburn
- ulcers
- gastroesophageal reflux disorder (GERD)
- irritable bowel syndrome (IBS)
- diverticulitis
- Crohn's disease (which causes ulcers to form in the gastrointestinal tract)
- digestive system cancer (Colorectal is the second leading cause of cancer in the United States.)

The Western diet, with its highly processed and chemicalized foods, is full of toxins and lacking in nutrients. It is high in proinflammatory sub-stances such as gluten and sugar, which increase acidity in the body and alter the gut terrain to create an ideal breeding ground for pathogenic bacteria to thrive. Fermented foods can enhance your digestive health by improving the internal terrain for beneficial microflora to thrive. When everything's in check, you increase the nutrients your body absorbs from the foods you eat.

So, where's the connection? How does a weak gut lead to a weak immune system—and hence, illness? As noted earlier, the human gastrointesti-nal tract houses the bulk of the human immune system. Everything you eat and drink will either strengthen or weaken your digestive system, which in turn affects your immune system. When you eat foods that are nutritionally deficient, the body is made weaker, not stronger, by making it easier for pathogenic organisms to invade the body and establish themselves. When you eat foods that contain toxic chemicals and harmful substances, as many junk foods do, your im-mune system reacts by creating an inflammatory response. It may also make antibodies against the toxins and harmful substances as though they were a foreign invader. When this occurs, your immune system has mobilized to finish the job of incomplete digestion but places unneeded stress on it. This also slows recovery and convalescence from illness.

When digestion becomes damaged or blocked, the health of all our cells is compromised. Over time, this can lead to other medical problems, such as arthritis, autoimmune disease, chronic fatigue, food sensitivities, and a variety of skin conditions (psoriasis and eczema), all of which—believe it or not—are digestive in origin. An acute symptom, such as heartburn or constipation, when left uncontrolled can cascade and develop into a chronic condition, such as inflammatory bowel disorder or candida overgrowth. Internally, the friendly bacteria help extract more nutrients from the foods we eat, produce trace minerals and vitamins, and protect us from harmful bacteria that may make us sick. If there is an imbalance in your intestinal flora, meaning that you have more harmful than friendly bacteria guarding the fort that is your immune system, then you are more likely to get sick. Your body's immune system defenses are reduced significantly without a healthy and abundant supply of these friendly bacterial microflora—microflora you can get by eating fermented foods. Improving the health of the digestive system, then, will improve the health of the immune system.

THE DARK SIDE OF ANTIBIOTICS, PASTEURIZATION, AND STERILIZATION

As a modern society, we've come to believe that antibiotics, pasteurization, and sterilization are the saviors of our health, but in reality they bring with them a threat—a dark side that rarely gets exposed. Beneficial bacteria in the gut have a direct influence on the immune system and are your first line of defense against infectious agents and sickness. Antibiotics are indiscriminate destroyers of all bacteria in the human body, including the beneficial bacteria that are not only in the gut but also in other organs and tissues. Further, for the past fifty or so years we've been waging an all-out war against germs, a war that includes sterilization and pasteurization. In our efforts to destroy bacteria, we've created more virulent strains that have become resistant to our weapons. While no one can argue the fact that antibiotics have saved countless lives, and that sterilization and pasteurization have their place, this war on germs has yet to show signs of relenting. And as with any war, there are casualties. The casualties, however, are often the patients, not just the germs. Fortunately, there are solutions, and fermented foods have much they can offer us to bolster our defenses.

Anti-Antibiotics

Within a population of healthy adults, the composition of gastrointestinal bacteria is relatively stable over time. Diet, disease, and the environment, however, can each influence the bacterial balance. Shifts in these variables that affect the continuity of our gut's microflora can serve as threats to our health. For example, when we take antibiotics to kill off infectious bacteria, we also destroy large amounts of the beneficial flora. When good gut bacteria are killed off, it can severely impair digestion and absorption of nutrients at a time when your body needs them most.

The word "antibiotic" comes from the Greek, *anti*, meaning "against," and *bios*, meaning "life." Antibiotics are chemical compounds that are themselves derived from microbes. But because they're unable to seek and destroy specific pathogens, antibiotics do collateral damage to good microbes in our bodies. In addition, research shows that antibiotics also mutate beneficial bacteria, which gain resistance to antibiotics, inspiring a vicious cycle of the need for stronger antibiotics that again leads to increased resistance. This is how we end up creating super bacteria, such as multi-drug resistant tuberculosis, staph, and strep.

Ultimately, repeated and unnecessary use of antibiotics weakens our immune systems. Numerous studies have confirmed that consistent use of antibiotics increases the population of antibiotic-resistant genes within the microbiome. While some good bacteria are killed along with the bad when you take an antibiotic, some bacteria, and all yeasts, are left unharmed. This changes the microflora balance and opens the door to an overgrowth of yeasts. One species of yeasts, *Candida albicans*, colonize rapidly, especially in your intestines and other parts of your digestive tract, where they contribute to a vast majority of diseases and infections. Direct consequences of yeast overgrowth from just one course of antibiotics can often include a number of common side effects such as diarrhea, vaginal yeast infections, and oral thrush. In most cases, these side effects go away within a short time once the antibiotics are discontinued and the microflora recovers its normal balance.

Another antibiotic that can change the normal balance of microflora is penicillin, which damages both *Lactobacilli* and *Bifidobacteria*, while promoting the growth of pathogenic bacteria. *Lactobacilli* are the only elements in the body that keep candida and other harmful yeast infections under control, so as these bacteria are destroyed whenever you take a course of antibiotics, candida spread like wildfire throughout your system.

The Cost of Hidden Antibiotics

It is not only antibiotics we take by prescription that we need to worry about, but also those we unintentionally consume with our food, because farmers use antibiotics when raising animals. Most commercially bred dairy cows are fed antibiotics to combat their unnatural, cramped living conditions. These antibiotics contribute to deadly infections such as E. coli, as well as mastitis brought on from excessive milk production. Studies have shown that these antibiotics leach into the cows' milk supplies and are then passed on to us. Antibiotics are even sprayed on fruits and vegetables to stave off disease but then end up in our bodies when we eat the food.

A primary effect of candida is suppression of the immune system, which means that the very drug you are taking to combat disease is impairing your only natural defense against it, both immediately and in the future. So effectively, an intestinal tract devoid of proper friendly intestinal bacteria is a breeding ground for future illness.

A final example is tetracyclines, antibiotics commonly used to treat acne and rosacea. These do not actually kill bacteria, but rather they prevent bacteria from growing, including the beneficial bacteria. Tetracyclines hurt the integrity of the gut wall, making it more susceptible to infection, and engage the immune system to attack itself, resulting in an autoimmune effect. Meanwhile, they facilitate detrimental fungus and bacterial growth in the intestinal tract, which can result in candida.

Because the use of antibiotics is necessary during certain disease conditions, it is crucial to replenish the body with probiotics and good microorganisms. Fortunately, consuming fermented foods will actively replenish your intestinal bacteria during and after a dose of antibiotics. Fermented foods rapidly return the normal microflora to its balance as their rich supply of probiotics reduces levels of certain harmful bacteria and yeasts through a natural process of competition. Daily consumption of fermented foods ensures a high number of immune-boosting microflora and promotes probiotic growth. Conversely, a poor diet, such as one high in sugar, which yeasts and bacteria thrive on, or any diet that does not contain probiotics, indirectly contributes to the recurrence of future health problems.

Pass on Pasteurization

Ever since its commercial use began in the 1920s, pasteurization has become a controversial topic. Pasteurization, the process of heating milk or other liquids to destroy microorganisms that can cause disease, kills the friendly bacteria along with the pathogenic.

The fermentation of milk illustrates the delicate balance between microbes and human intervention. When unpasteurized, or raw, milk is left unrefrigerated for a period, it turns sour because of the growth of *Lactobacilli*. When this sour milk is used to prepare bread, it creates a special sour taste and increases the softness of the dough. Pasteurized milk, on the other hand, is devoid of all microorganisms, and when left without refrigeration, it spoils due to the growth of undesirable bacteria.

Ultra-pasteurization, which takes milk from a chilled temperature to above the boiling point in less than two seconds, is even more detrimental than standard pasteurization methods. While this process gives milk a longer shelf life, it alters casein (the protein found in milk) and is believed to be one of the factors creating rising rates of casein sensitivity. Most commercially produced dairy products are pasteurized, which destroys beneficial probiotics and enzymes. Raw milk and fermented dairy products, such as yogurt and kefir, are better choices because these are enzyme rich and contain the probiotics that restore friendly microflora.

Similar to pasteurization, irradiation of food has become standard practice in the United States and other parts of the world. The controversial process is a relative newcomer among food-preserving techniques and is used on fruits, vegetables, wheat flour, beef, pork, poultry, eggs, spices, and herb teas. During irradiation, food is exposed to ionizing radiation in an effort to destroy microorganisms, viruses, or insects that could be dangerous if consumed. Irradiation can also be used to prevent sprouting or delay ripening. For example, strawberries that are irradiated can last for up to two weeks, compared to less than one week for untreated berries.

The process of irradiation damages the DNA of the food to stunt its further growth. Depending on the dose of irradiation and the storage time, irradiated foods can lose from 5 to 80 percent of many important nutrients, including vitamins A, B complex, C, E, and K. Currently, there have not been enough studies performed to determine all the effects of irradiation on foods, but because it reduces a food's nutrient value, it makes sense to select locally grown or organic foods, which will not have been irradiated.

Sterilization Used to Disinfect

A 1996 University of Texas study conducted on germ-free, or sterile, animals revealed the extent of dependence on the normal microflora for the body's defense system and for digestion. In the study, the growth and development of animals reared under normal conditions were compared with test animals that were delivered via Caesarean section and raised in an environment completely free of germs to ensure that they would not come into contact with normal microflora. Researchers observed that the germ-free animals were different physiologically as well as anatomically than the animals that contained the normal microflora. The germ-free animals did not have well-developed intestines and had a relative inability to digest food. Additionally, the lack of normal microflora led to a poor defense mechanism in these animals.

The Texas study helps us understand the relevance of the normal microflora in the human body and their significance in the normal functioning of the body. Though this research is still at an early stage, preliminary findings are encouraging.

The Hidden Cost of "Clean" Food

Food sterilization, in the form of irradiation and pasteurization, inevitably has a negative impact on the function of your body's digestive system. Food is often sterilized in order to extend the shelf life of many processed foods, as well as to kill any potential pests present on fruits and vegetables. However, this process will also decrease the diversity of microflora you consume by destroying the good bacteria that maintain the balance of your gut microflora.

THE IMPORTANCE OF PREBIOTICS

In addition to eating probiotic-rich fermented foods, you need to provide a congenial internal environment for the probiotic microbes to be produced and to multiply. Certain foods we select—called prebiotics—provide nutrients and create a compatible terrain for probiotic microbes to thrive. Dietary fiber is the best known prebiotic. While your body can't fully digest fiber and turn it into fuel, probiotic microbes can. Prebiotics are carbohydrates such as sugar and starch and are found in all foods of plant origin. Because humans do not have the necessary enzymes to break down these specific types of carbohydrates into smaller pieces that can be absorbed by the gut, they are available as a source of fuel for the beneficial bacteria in the large bowel. In this way, prebiotics help discourage the growth and activity of harmful bacteria by selectively increasing the numbers of beneficial bacteria.

There are two main types of fiber, contained within certain plants, that act as prebiotics: inulin and fructooligosaccharide (FOS). The term "oligosaccharide" refers to a short chain of sugar molecules from the Greek *oligo*, meaning "few" and *sacchar*, meaning "sugar." We can't digest these fibers, but probiotic microbes can. The main plants containing FOS and inulin are leeks, onions, garlic, asparagus, Jerusalem artichoke, chicory root, endive, radicchio, burdock, bananas, and dandelions. Prebiotics not only feed healthy bacteria but will also increase bioavailability of certain minerals in these foods. In addition, prebiotics help support natural immune defenses of the gut such as secretory immunoglobulin A (sIgA), the antibody naturally produced by the body to protect mucosal surfaces against infectious organisms and toxins. Working together, this "biotics" team is what keeps your digestive system working properly.

Adding fiber to your daily diet is essential for digestive health. Dietary fiber provides relief from symptoms such as irritable bowel syndrome, chronic abdominal pain, and various other inflammatory conditions in the gastrointestinal tract. If you're not accustomed to eating lots of fiber, you'll want to add these foods gradually, to give your body time to adjust. (Too much fiber at one time may cause temporary discomfort from symptoms such as bloating or gas.) And as you increase your fiber intake, be sure to also increase your hydration by drinking more water. The bottom line is that inulin and fructooligosaccharides boost intestinal flora and need to be a regular part of the diet to ensure optimum health.

OPTIMAL BALANCE IS WITHIN YOU

As you can see, our inner ecosystem is much like a rainforest with a very complex web of life. We house a variety of beneficial microbes that rely on us as much as we rely on them for nourishment and health. Keeping this delicate balance in harmony by avoiding overgrowth of any harmful species is indeed a worthwhile goal. In the next chapter we'll look at the therapeutic value of fermented foods and discuss various disease conditions that can be helped by daily consumption of them.

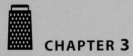

CHAPTER 3

How Fermented Foods Support Good Health

"All diseases begin in the gut."

— HIPPOCRATES

For thousands of years, people around the world have fermented foods as a way to preserve them and for their nutritional and therapeutic value. Including fermented foods in your daily diet supports health and vitality.

Here is a summary of their benefits:

- They crowd out pathogenic bacteria, candida, and parasites and provide life-supporting probiotics to strengthen your immune system.
- They increase enzyme production, thereby improving the digestive tract's ability to absorb and use food and nutrients.
- They enhance nutritional value in food, resulting in increased amounts of vitamins and minerals.
- They balance the body's overall pH, creating a more alkaline blood as well as an acidic environment in your stomach, which kills pathogens and is conducive for digestive system health.

The right nutrition can help your body not only heal itself but also possibly even reverse chronic disease, and the beneficial flora in fermented foods substantially contribute to this goal. The action of probiotic microorganisms during the preparation and process of fermenting food improves the quantity, availability, and digestibility of many essential dietary nutrients. The type and number of the gut bacteria plays an important role in determining health and disease in the human body. But in order to protect intestinal and immune function, your body must maintain an ecological balance of bacteria. If harmful bacteria are given the upper hand in this delicate balance, the door opens to infections, disease, and allergic reactions. Processed and chemicalized foods, environmental pollutants, stress, and long courses of antibiotics upset the balance and provide bad bugs with the ideal breeding ground, resulting in diminished digestion and compromised immunity.

Fortunately, there are actions you can take to handle modern living's damaging effects on your system—and fermented foods hold many of the solutions. A number of studies in humans and animals suggest lactic acid–producing microflora can inhibit the incidence, duration, and severity of some degenerative diseases and improve immune system function. In this chapter we'll discuss the nutritional and therapeutic value of fermented foods and look at how they may benefit, or in some cases prevent, several of these disease conditions.

IMMUNE-BOOSTING EFFECTS OF FERMENTED FOODS

Every day your body is bombarded by bacteria. And every day it's the job of your immune system to protect you from them. Many of us take our immune system for granted or may think that we're invincible—that is, until it stops performing optimally, and we get sick. But your immune system is not so different from a car. If you don't take proper care of it, it won't perform as well. The same is true with your immune system. The beneficial bacteria in fermented foods are the "oil" that helps you maintain your immune system engine.

Your immune system comprises both a protective and a responsive component that play vital interacting roles in health maintenance—both in regulating and in stimulating the body's responses to foreign invaders. The protective component, called the innate (or nonspecific) immune system, is made up of physical barriers that prevent pathogens from entering the body. Digestive, respiratory, urinary, and reproductive tracts are part of these barriers, and they are all lined with mucous membranes. If the barrier is weak, pathogens slip right through and an adaptive immune response takes over by engaging the natural killer cells to hunt down and kill the attackers. If the enemy attackers get past this first line of defense, your immune system responds with deeper attack against the pathogens. This is the immune system's responsive component known as the acquired (or specific) immune system, when the white blood cells produce specific antibodies, both T cells and B cells, that neutralize such attackers. The best defense is a good offense, and as we saw in chapter 2, your best strategy is to consume fermented foods on a daily basis.

A number of studies have showcased the immune-boosting effects of probiotics from fermented foods. The majority of evidence from in vitro studies on both animals and humans show that beneficial bacteria enhance mucus production through stimulation of secretory IgA, which protects the mucosal barrier lining the gut wall and thereby defends against invasion and colonization by pathogenic microorganisms. The secretory IgA system serves as a first line of immune defense, and any threat to the proper functioning of the mucosal barrier brings the risk of serious disease. Beneficial bacteria also enhance white blood cell counts, thus enabling an efficient immune response to pathogens. Probiotics also increase macrophage activity, natural killer cells, and immunoglobulins, which further promote the protection of the immune barrier. When several strains of lactic acid bacteria, such as *Lactobacillus acidophilus*, *Lactobacillus rhamnosus*, and *Bifidobacterium lactis*, are consumed together, they work synergistically and may further enhance the immune response.

Several studies have suggested probiotics can be useful in combating inflammatory-type diseases, because of their potential for regulating the immune system. Such areas of study include the following findings:

- The immune system plays an essential role in the modification of inflammatory-type diseases such as inflammatory bowel disease (IBD) and Crohn's disease, and consequently a dysfunction of the immune system can lead to exacerbation of such diseases.

- A study on allergy-related responses, such as food intolerance and nasal allergies, demonstrated decreased allergic responses in allergen-sensitized mice after they were given strains of *Lactobacilli* orally.

- One study demonstrated probiotics' usefulness in combating juvenile chronic arthritis. Although the mechanism for this was uncertain, it is believed that by increasing immune-signaling events of the gut microflora, immune-stimulating activity was also enhanced.

- Another study showed lacto bacterial organisms were effective in reducing the symptoms of inflammatory bowel disease, such as a reduction of abdominal pain, a decrease in gastrointestinal inflammation and permeability (leaky gut), and the alleviation of bloating, flatulence, and constipation.

Can Fermented Food Be Medicine?

Hippocrates, the father of modern medicine, said more than twenty-five hundred years ago, "Let food be thy medicine, and medicine be thy food." It is through our food and nutrition that we create the right environment that sets the foundation for good health to occur. The body requires fifty essential vitamins and minerals each day to sustain optimal health, and it derives these almost entirely from food. Eating fermented foods increases the supply of nutrients and enhances the absorption of these nutrients in the body.

Probiotics also boost immune function in people whose immune systems are not functioning optimally. Studies have demonstrated that malnourished children and infants sensitive to allergens, which can occur as a result of exposure to high levels of antigens during early infancy, have improved after being given *Lactobacillus*. At the other end of the age spectrum, probiotics have proven useful in boosting the functioning of the immune system at the cellular level in elderly subjects.

Because 70 to 80 percent of the immune system is located in and around the gut, if you have digestive system problems you are more susceptible to having a weakened immune system. Ultimately, your diet impacts your gut microflora, but stress can also damage the gastrointestinal microflora. Long-term stress of any kind may result in permanent damage to beneficial flora. It will be almost impossible to permanently eliminate distress symptoms unless you improve the balance between the beneficial bacteria and the disease-causing bacteria that exist naturally in your gastrointestinal tract. It makes good sense to fine-tune and strengthen this area with probiotic-rich fermented foods.

NUTRITIONAL VALUE OF FERMENTED FOODS

A significant body of research credits the beneficial and therapeutic effects of consuming fermented foods and probiotics. Classified as Generally Recognized as Safe (GRAS) by the U.S. Food and Drug Administration, the process of fermentation increases the potency of many vitamins, minerals, and enzymes. This is due mainly to the friendly bacteria that partially digest the food, making the nutrients inside more bioavailable and easier for your body to absorb. As a result, we gain more vitamins and minerals from fermented foods than we do from cooked or raw unfermented foods.

The Value of Vitamins

Vitamins are considered micronutrients that are essential to life because the body needs them in small amounts to perform important functions, such as regulating metabolism and assisting the biochemical processes that release energy from digested food. Fermentation enables certain microorganisms to produce these essential vitamins at a higher rate than your body would do without them. The main vitamins that get a boost through fermentation are C, B complex, A, and K.

Foods Rich in Vitamin C

Cabbage, beets, tomatoes, collards, kale, turnips, peppers, onions, plums, papayas, cherries, pineapples, citrus fruits, strawberries, raspberries, blueberries, kiwifruit, cantaloupe, Brussels sprouts, cauliflower, and carrots are all excellent food choices high in vitamin C.

Consider vitamin C, for example. The body requires this essential vitamin on a daily basis for hundreds of metabolic functions. It is a powerful antioxidant that helps retard the aging process of cells and boosts the immune system by stimulating both the production and the function of leukocytes (white blood cells). Additionally, vitamin C is required for, or plays an essential role, in the following processes:

- synthesizing collagen, an important structural component of blood vessels, tendons, ligaments, and bone

- synthesizing the neurotransmitter norepinephrine, which is critical to brain function and is known to affect mood

- metabolizing cholesterol, which may have implications for blood cholesterol levels and the incidence of gallstones

- increasing cardioprotective capabilities by improving blood flow through coronary arteries

- promoting healing of all cells, allowing us to better deal with both external and internal stressors and reducing risk for certain diseases such as scurvy, atherosclerosis and coronary artery disease, stroke, gout, cataracts, hypertension, diabetes, cancer, and even the common cold

- supporting the good gut bacteria and destroying harmful bacteria and viruses

- protecting cells and their DNA from damage and mutation, which helps support the body's immune system, thereby increasing the body's ability to prevent certain cancer-causing compounds from forming

Because our bodies do not have the ability to make their own vitamin C, we must obtain it through our diet. All fermented vegetables and fruits contain massive amounts of vitamin C, but we will absorb up to three or possibly four hundred times more vitamin C from, for example, fermented cabbage as sauerkraut than from cooked or raw cabbage.

Foods Rich in Vitamins A and K

Fish liver oils, animal livers, apricots, asparagus, beet greens, broccoli, carrots, cantaloupe, collards, dandelion greens, dulse, kale, garlic, mustard greens, papayas, peaches, pumpkin, red peppers, spinach, spirulina, sweet potatoes, turnip, Swiss chard, and yellow squash are all excellent food choices high in vitamin A.

Asparagus, blackstrap molasses, broccoli, Brussels sprouts, cabbage, cauliflower, dark green leafy vegetables, egg yolks, leaf lettuce, liver, oatmeal, oats, rye, soybeans, wheat, and yogurt are all excellent food choices high in vitamin K.

Friendly flora help manufacture several other essential vitamins, including the B-complex vitamins—thiamin (B1), riboflavin (B2), niacin (B3), pantothenic acid (B5), pyridoxine (B6), cobalamin (B12), biotin, and folic acid. These vitamins help produce energy and maintain cellular functions. Each member of the B complex has a unique structure and performs a distinct function in the body:

- B5 and B6 help fight infection to protect the body against disease.

- B2, B3, B5, B6, and biotin convert glucose into energy. A deficiency of any of these vitamins leads to lethargy and fatigue.

- B12 helps reduce or eliminate anemia.

- B1, B6, and folate lower the risk of heart disease.

- B5, B6, and B12 minimize or even eliminate depression.

- B1 is essential for proper digestion and production of hydrochloric acid in the stomach, where they assist in the metabolism of proteins, fats, and carbohydrates.

- B5 is necessary for healthy functioning of the entire nervous system; it aids in the correct functioning of the adrenal glands as well as the production of some hormones and nerve-regulating substances.

- B5 is chiefly responsible for releasing hormones in response to stress through the synthesis of corticosteroids such as cortisol and epinephrine.

All B vitamins are water soluble, meaning that the body does not store them. Therefore, it is of utmost importance that our daily diet provide the nutrients necessary for us to make them. Because of their ability to manufacture the full complex of B vitamins, the beneficial flora in fermented foods do just that.

Fermented foods also contain high amounts of vitamin A, a group of fat-soluble retinoids, including retinol, and retinoic acid. Vitamin A and its counterparts are involved in immune function, night vision, reproduction, bone growth, and cellular communication. It acts as an antioxidant and plays a critical role in the immune system by helping make white blood cells, which fight off viruses and harmful bacteria. Vitamin A is essential for the health and maintenance of the heart, lungs, kidneys, and other vital organs.

Fermented foods are also rich in the antioxidant vitamin K. It plays a key role in keeping calcium in the bones from migrating into the arteries, thus helping to prevent atherosclerosis. It is an essential nutrient necessary for blood clotting and plays an important role in blood sugar regulation, which helps with prevention or management of diabetes.

Foods Rich in B-Complex Vitamins

Brown rice, oatmeal, egg yolks, legumes, rice bran, wheat bran, whole grains, peas, port, broccoli, Brussels sprouts, asparagus, brewer's yeast, liver, peanuts, pork, poultry, dulse, kelp, spirulina, raisins, plums, dried prunes, most nuts, and watercress are all excellent choices that are high in B-complex vitamins.

The Significance of Minerals

Minerals are naturally occurring substances that your body requires for proper function and structure. There are two main groups of minerals: macro-minerals (calcium, magnesium, sodium, potassium, and phosphorus) and micro-minerals, also known as trace minerals (copper, selenium, silicon, iodine, chromium, iron, manganese, boron, and zinc).

Fermentation increases certain minerals like calcium, which is critical for strong bones and teeth, heart, and nervous system function, and muscle growth and contraction. Calcium is found mostly in dairy products, salmon, sardines, sesame seeds, oats, and dark green leafy vegetables, but it is made more available for uptake in the body through fermented dairy products.

Zinc is another mineral that is increased through the fermentation of legumes such as soybeans. Zinc is vital for a healthy immune system, wound healing, prostate gland function in men, and the growth of reproductive organs in both men and women. Zinc is found in kelp, dulse, legumes, soybeans, lima beans, sunflower seeds, mushrooms, brewer's yeast, and whole grains.

Augment Antioxidants

Large amounts of antioxidants in fermented foods help keep free radicals in check. Free radicals are single atoms of oxygen that are highly reactive and are produced by every cell of the body as an end product of metabolism. The molecules can also come to us from the environment, but they can still damage cells through their interactions with oxygen. The free oxygen atoms that are in a highly reactive state act on the DNA of cells, leading to mutations. Extensive DNA mutations by these free radicals lead to uncontrolled cell division that is witnessed in cancer or the kind of cell death seen in aging. The presence of antioxidants, particularly vitamin C, found in fermented vegetables and soy foods, has been shown to significantly reduce oxidative stress by neutralizing free radicals. The benefits of reducing oxidative stress may enhance longevity and even protect the body from developing cancer. Fermentation increases the level of antioxidants in food (lycopene in tomatoes, resveratrol in grapes, vitamin C in cabbage, and beta-carotene in carrots), as well as increases antioxidant enzymes that are made by the body.

Enzymes, the Miracle Workers

In addition to beneficial microorganisms, fermented foods are loaded with enzymes that are necessary for every chemical reaction that takes place in the human body, thus making life possible. Enzymes help build our bodies from proteins, fats, and carbohydrates, and without them, our bodies could not utilize vitamins or minerals from food. They help break down food into simpler components that can be absorbed by the body; most foods require specific enzymes to liberate their nutritional potential. There are three main types of enzymes:

- **Metabolic enzymes** run our bodies, including maintaining the health of our organs and tissues, and their main job is to keep everything working properly.

- **Digestive enzymes** are responsible for digesting protein, fat, and carbohydrates and breaking them down into components that can be absorbed into the bloodstream and carried throughout the body.

- **Food enzymes** from raw foods start food digestion and help the digestive enzymes run more efficiently.

Enzymes' efforts, however, can be thwarted when your diet contains heavily processed, sugary foods that deplete your body's ability to make enzymes. Unfortunately, fragile enzymes get denatured, or inactivated, at high temperatures (above 106°F [41°C]). When the diet consists of too many cooked foods and not enough raw foods, metabolic enzymes are called in to help digest food rather than run your metabolism and organs. Apart from slowing down the works, this can pose all sorts of problems to your metabolism. A less efficient metabolism and a weakened immune system could make you more susceptible to both acute conditions, such as bacterial infections, and chronic degenerative conditions, such as arthritis and asthma, and could potentially be a contributing factor in cancer.

Enzyme deficiency caused by the standard America diet will ultimately lead to poor digestion and diminished nutrient absorption, causing constipation, bloating, cramps, flatulence, heartburn, and acid reflux. Your body produces only a finite amount of enzymes in a lifetime, and this production slows down with aging. The lack of digestive enzymes caused by aging and poor diet gives rise to poor health. Over time, a diet that is poor in enzyme-rich, raw, live foods depletes the body's supply of digestive and metabolic enzymes. Fortunately, the enzymes found in fermented foods can help replenish enzymes and restore digestion. It's essential that you consume adequate amounts of foods that contain enzymes. Raw fermented foods are the answer: they are extremely rich in enzymes and are an effective and efficient way to rebuild your digestive system and replenish your supply of enzymes.

Fermented foods, particularly vegetables and fruits, which are rich in digestive enzymes, can help improve digestive processes. By supporting the increased absorption of nutrients, enzymes ultimately provide you with increased energy levels and reduce the effort exerted by your body toward digestion. Your metabolic enzymes are spared the task of digesting food and can return instead to their normal job of keeping your metabolism and organs running smoothly.

DISEASES HELPED BY FERMENTED FOODS

In a world where fast foods, anti-nutrients, oxidized fats, denatured proteins, enzyme destruction, and vitamin- and mineral-depleted foods have become the standard by which we evaluate our nutritional choices, the best options for a healthy and long life can be daunting. Fortunately, fermented foods' natural antibiotic, health-building, and disease-preventive qualities provide a path through the confusion into a harmonious union of both nutrition and medicine.

As we've seen, probiotics improve digestive-system and immune-system function. They've been found to reverse some diseases and prevent others. A growing body of evidence confirms that certain probiotic strains of *Lactobacilli* are able to control a number of chronic diseases ranging from obesity, cardiovascular disease, and hypertension to autoimmune diseases such as rheumatoid arthritis, multiple sclerosis, and diabetes, and from immune dysfunction diseases such as HIV and even cancer to psychological conditions. We may not fully understand the mechanism by which each of these diseases is ameliorated; however, we do know these bacteria strengthen the body's army of antibodies to help combat all these diseases.

Dr. Elie Metchnikoff first presented the concept of probiotics in his 1907 book, *The Prolongation of Life*, written from the Pasteur Institute Lab in Paris. He discovered that fermented milks reversed the decomposition of gut microflora. After noticing that Bulgarians had longer life spans, he carefully studied their lifestyle which revealed that they consumed fermented milk as part of their regular diet. This landmark study brought to the fore the importance of probiotics and the benefits of fermented food to health.

A Friendly Yeast

Another type of probiotic, a yeast called Saccharomyces boulardii, *is not part of the naturally occurring gut flora. It has, however, been shown to have numerous health benefits, including clearing the skin and controlling diarrhea caused by antibiotics. Although yeasts make up only 0.1 percent of the gut flora, they are ten times larger in size than bacteria and can cause imbalances in the bacterial levels. S. boulardii enhances levels of gut secretory IgA and inhibits the growth of the pathogenic yeast* Candida albicans *by producing lactic and other acids. It has also been used effectively in people with Crohn's disease by supporting growth of beneficial bacteria and significantly reducing the number of bowel movements. Fermented foods help create an ideal breeding ground for these friendly helpers.*

Most probiotics fall into the group of organisms known as lactic acid–producing bacteria, which help acidify the intestinal tract and protect us from overgrowth of harmful bacteria. Research validates that the lactic acid produced from beneficial bacteria can decrease the incidence, duration, and severity of these gastrointestinal illnesses:

- inflammatory bowel disorders, including inflammatory bowel disease (IBD), small intestinal bacterial overgrowth (SIBO), and ulcerative colitis
- celiac disease
- peptic ulcers
- *Helicobacter pylori* infections
- irritable bowel syndrome (IBS)
- viral gastroenteritis
- antibiotic-associated diarrhea
- traveler's diarrhea
- stomach flu
- lactose intolerance
- infant's colic

The magic of fermentation lies in how it makes it easy for your digestive system to gain maximum benefits from foods, and fermentation is especially powerful in helping heal digestive system disorders. The beneficial microorganisms help lay the foundation that provides the right environment for optimal digestion to occur. Let's take a closer look at a few of the digestive complaints that can be alleviated by eating and drinking fermented foods.

Chronic Gastritis

This is a condition that includes inflammation or irritation of the lining of the stomach, caused by a number of factors that include stress and infection by *Helicobacter* species, a bacteria that has been implicated in gastric and duodenal ulcers. It affects 80 percent of the population worldwide. A 2010 study published in *World Journal of Gastroenterology* investigated the therapeutic effect of milk fermented with *Streptococcus thermophilus* on chronic gastritis. They found that the fermented milk was able to return the gastric mucosa to healthy levels. Furthermore, the effectiveness was similar to that of a commercial drug commonly used in the treatment of gastritis.

Lactose Intolerance

Lactose intolerance affects an estimated 75 percent of adults worldwide. Many people become increasingly lactose intolerant as they grow older, generally because the body stops producing lactase, a milk sugar–digesting enzyme, after a child is weaned off mother's milk. Lactose is a sugar, commonly referred to as milk sugar, that is present in dairy foods and causes stomach cramps, gas, bloating, diarrhea, and sometimes nausea in people who cannot digest it. Studies have shown that it's possible to control—and in some cases, eliminate symptoms of—lactose intolerance by eating yogurt that is rich in *Bifidobacterium bifidis* or *Lactobacillus bulgaricus*, two bacteria that ferment lactose. These bacteria convert the lactose into lactic acid, resulting in a product that is more easily digestible.

Milk: It Does a Gut Good

A 2010 study on the effects of milk fermented with Lactobacillus casei *on the degree of illness among kids between three and six years old found that there was a decrease in the rate of common infectious diseases among the kids who drank the special milk. In addition to the decreased severity of the illnesses, which was 19 percent lower than that of the control group, researchers found that there was a drastic reduction in the number of gastrointestinal diseases among those kids who drank the fermented milk.*

Crohn's Disease

Crohn's disease is an inflammatory bowel disorder that usually affects the lowest portion of the small intestine, but it can occur in other parts of the digestive tract, from the mouth to the anus. It affects men and women equally and tends to run in families. Researchers believe that Crohn's disease has a genetic basis, but that it doesn't appear until triggered by the presence of bacteria or a virus that provokes an abnormal activation of the immune system.

In a 2008 French study conducted on Crohn's disease patients, researchers found a decrease in the abundance and biodiversity of intestinal bacteria within the dominant phylum, Firmicutes. Scientists observed that a reduction of a major member of Firmicutes, *F. prausnitzii*, is associated with a higher risk of recurrence of Crohn's disease. In subsequent studies they found that *F. prausnitzii* led to significantly lower proinflammatory cytokines and exhibited the highest anti-inflammatory profile. Though it didn't kill bad bacteria, the results of orally administered *F. prausnitzii* suggest counterbalancing effects on dysbiosis and is a promising probiotic strategy in Crohn's disease treatment.

A well-balanced gut microflora with a strong population of probiotic bacteria goes a long way toward ensuring healthy functioning of the digestive tract. Feed and nurture your friendly bacteria in your body as you would a beloved pet. By keeping the bacteria inside you happy and in balance, so, too, does this guarantee a healthier, happier you!

Apart from gastrointestinal disorders, there are a variety of proposed beneficial health effects of probiotics in other chronic health conditions. Numerous clinical studies conducted over the years confirm that probiotics can bring relief to patients with physically and emotionally debilitating symptoms. Many of these disease conditions have overlapping symptoms with an immune system connection. Because the digestive system houses the bulk of your immune system, it makes sense to strengthen this area with therapeutic doses of beneficial flora by consuming probiotics and fermented foods. Research into the causality and effectiveness of probiotics on many of these conditions is in its infancy, but a probiotic case can be made for each of the following chronic conditions.

Allergic Diseases

There are strong connections between allergic diseases (including rhinitis, hay fever, and food sensitivities) and microbial activity. Probiotics serve to boost immunity and prevent colonization of pathogenic bacteria. Studies have shown that infants receiving *Lactobacillus GG* in their formula showed significant improvement against inflammatory allergic disorders such as food sensitivities and rhinitis.

Asthma

Changes in gut microflora can cause vulnerability to food and environmental allergies and bring on attacks of asthma. Probiotics help the immune system develop regulatory T cells, which can help turn off inflammation throughout the body and improve immune function.

Autism

Probiotics help eliminate toxins from the body and restore gut wall integrity to enhance digestive system and immune system function. Studies are showing that children and adults with autism often have higher amounts of gut pathogens and have more gastrointestinal problems.

Autoimmune Diseases

Autoimmune diseases (rheumatoid arthritis, multiple sclerosis, psoriasis, lupus, type 1 diabetes, Grave's disease, Hashimoto's disease, Guillain-Barre syndrome, scleroderma, and Sjogren's syndrome) have definite digestive system components. There are usually inflammation and malabsorption issues, and small bowel bacterial overgrowth is common. Probiotics can help reduce toxins and rebalance the gut microflora to reduce infectious agents. Let's examine a few of these conditions helped by bacteria.

Rheumatoid Arthritis

Approximately 350 million people worldwide suffer from arthritis. It is the most common cause of disability in the United States, striking one in five adults and limiting the ability of nearly 21 million people. Arthritis is the inflammation of one or more joints and is characterized by pain and stiffness, swelling, deformity, and a diminished range of motion. Supplemental probiotics and the fermented foods that contain them have proven to be effective in reducing inflammation associated with rheumatic arthritis. Probiotics help through modulation of inflammatory responses, directly in the gastrointestinal tract and indirectly in the immune system.

In a 1997 study conducted in Finland, researchers tested the effect of dietary therapy with *Lactobacillus GG* or bovine colostrum on thirty patients with juvenile arthritis for two weeks. The researchers observed that gut defense mechanisms are disturbed in chronic juvenile arthritis, which exerts a direct effect on immune system responses. The probiotics showed potential to reinforce the mucosal barrier mechanisms in this disorder, thus lowering inflammation. When inflamed, the gastrointestinal tract becomes permeable and can lead to dysbiosis and serves as a link between gastrointestinal inflammatory disorders and extra-inflammatory diseases such as arthritis. Probiotics have the ability to reduce such permeability and control allergic inflammation.

Multiple Sclerosis

Multiple sclerosis (MS) is a progressive, degenerative disease of the central nervous system, including the brain, spinal cord, and optic nerve. It affects an estimated 2.5 million people worldwide. Although the underlying cause of MS is not fully known, it is widely believed to be an autoimmune disease influenced by genetic and environmental factors. The symptoms may mysteriously occur and then disappear, and symptoms are often preceded by stress and poor nutrition. Poor nutrient absorption, food intolerances or allergies, and a buildup of toxins in the body also are important factors.

Biologists at California Institute of Technology suggest that microorganisms play a role in the onset or progression of the disease and that gut bacteria may be the missing environmental component. In 2010, the team of biologists conducted studies on mice to determine how profoundly gut microbes, both harmful and helpful, affect the immune system's inflammatory response and thus create conditions that could allow the disease symptoms of MS to develop. Interestingly, the study showed that specific bacteria in the intestines can affect the central nervous system during an attack of MS. The researchers concluded that when the composition of gut bacteria becomes imbalanced—say, from changes in the diet, stress, or antibiotic use—this can result in dysbiosis, which disrupts the balance between pro- and anti-inflammatory bacteria and leads to diseases like MS. These findings reveal that intestinal microflora profoundly affect the immune responses and suggest that probiotics and fermented foods may prove beneficial in a therapeutic program directed toward MS.

Diabetes

Mounting evidence suggests a relationship exists between gut microbiota and its role in obesity-related disorders, including insulin resistance and diabetes. Obesity studies conducted on mice fed high-fat, high-carbohydrate diets have identified several mechanisms at play. After four weeks of high-fat feeding, the mice exhibited obese characteristics, accompanied by an altered composition of the microbiota. These changes were totally reversed after a shift back to the original low-fat, low-carbohydrate diet. Other mechanisms linking gut microbiota to obesity-related disorders include chronic low-grade endotoxinemia, which occurs as a result of toxins that are released by bacteria after destruction of the bacterial cell wall, and changes in gut-derived peptide secretion.

Further, in a 2012 Chinese study, people with type 2 diabetes were found to have a moderate imbalance in gut bacteria, specifically lower levels of butyrate-producing bacteria. More studies need to be conducted connecting the relationship between gut microbes and diabetes, but the research is promising.

Blood Cholesterol and Hyperlipidemia

Probiotics, especially *L. acidophilus*, have been shown to reduce LDL (bad) cholesterol and triglycerides, through various mechanisms which may include binding to and preventing LDL from being released back into the bloodstream. More clinical research is needed.

Cardiovascular Disease and Hypertension

The World Health Organization estimates that coronary heart disease affects some 17 million people worldwide each year. Coronary heart disease, which is caused by a narrowing of the coronary arteries, is the most common form of heart disease and can lead to heart attacks and strokes. Preliminary evidence suggests that both prebiotics and probiotics are beneficial in lowering high blood cholesterol and the associated risk factors for atherosclerotic cardiovascular disease (a condition where the arteries become narrowed and hardened due to an excessive buildup of plaque). Several animal studies have demonstrated that lactic acid bacteria may lower blood cholesterol levels by breaking down bile in the gut, which enters the blood as cholesterol, thus inhibiting its reabsorption. Probiotics can reduce arterial inflammation (inflammation creates blockages) by supporting development of T cells that help reduce inflammatory responses throughout the body.

A variety of research published in the September 2009 issue of *International Journal of Molecular Sciences* found probiotics to be beneficial in the treatment of high blood pressure. The studies demonstrated the supporting role of probiotics in lowering blood cholesterol, specifically LDL, which subsequently leads to a reduced risk of hypertension that is often associated with coronary heart disease. In preliminary studies, elderly patients who consumed fermented milk with a starter containing *Lactobacillus helveticus* and *Saccharomyces cerevisiae* showed reductions in systolic and diastolic blood pressure. While additional research is needed, these preliminary studies are most encouraging.

Colorectal Cancer

There is evidence suggesting that probiotic bacteria might reduce cancer risk through several mechanisms. Probiotics alter the terrain of the intestine, thereby decreasing populations or metabolic activities of pathogenic bacteria that may generate carcinogens. They also stimulate growth of friendly bacteria to guard the immune system and better defend against cancer cell growth. Probiotics produce metabolic products that improve a cell's ability to die when it should die (a process known as apoptosis). Probiotics improve absorption and assimilation of proteins, vitamins, and minerals to increase healthy metabolism of the host. Additionally, they produce compounds that inhibit the growth of tumor cells. Finally, probiotics improve detoxification of ingested carcinogens.

 Molds Fight Cancer, Too

Japan is well known for its consumption of traditional fermented foods, Including rice wine (sake), distilled spirit (shochu), soy paste (miso), soy sauce (shoyu), and dried bonito (katsuobushi), which are all manufactured using molds such as Aspergillus and Eurotium. These molds have been used for manufacturing fermented foods for many years and are generally recognized as safe (GRAS). Molds also have been found to impart anticancer properties through fermented food. A 2010 study conducted at Nagoya University, in Japan, tested the antioxidant derivatives , produced by the molds used in fermented foods. In the study, they were found to inhibit tumor formation in mice. Specifically, they were shown to have high free radical–scavenger ability and exhibited tumor-inhibiting abilities.

To date, only animal studies have investigated the direct effects of probiotics on immune responses on cancer and tumor regression. The evidence accumulated thus far suggests that the health benefits probiotics confer are via modulation of immune system function. Enhancement of natural killer cell (NK) activity, T cell and B cell stimulation, and reduction of proinflammatory cytokines are a few of the mechanisms by which probiotics have been shown to improve immunity and to make the destruction of infected cells in the body more effective. So far, the animal studies directed at fighting various forms of gastrointestinal tract–related cancers are encouraging. Here are some examples:

- A 2012 study conducted at the University of North Carolina showed that orally administrated probiotics reduced the establishment and growth of colorectal cancer cells in mice. Growth of secondary tumors was also inhibited following tumor resection.

- A 2010 study conducted in the United Kingdom demonstrated that mice fed the *Lactobacillus casei* strain *Shirota* developed fewer systemic tumors while the comparative immune responses in non-probiotic-fed mice declined markedly during tumor development.

- A 2011 study conducted by the University of Halle, in Germany, demonstrated that fermented wheat germ extract contains naturally occurring substances that prevent the proliferation of colorectal cancer cells and cause cell apoptosis. The study showed that fermented wheat germ extract was also effective in reducing the chances of cancer reoccurrence.

- A 2012 study conducted by the Institute of Experimental Medicine, in Slovak Republic, demonstrated the protective effect of prebiotics on colon cancer in rats. The consumption of prebiotics increased the number of *Lactobacilli* in the stomach, which acted as the protective factor against colon cancer. (Prebiotics, which we discussed in chapter 2, increase levels of *Bifidobacteria* and *L. acidophilus* in the colon. When used along with probiotics from fermented foods, they aid and benefit the colon by creating an ideal breeding ground and crowding out bad bacteria.) The study showed there was an enhanced production of short-chain fatty acids, which boost the growth of *Lactobacilli* and *Bifidobacteria*.

- In another study, rats that were treated to yogurt fermented with *Lactobacillus delbrueckii* and *Streptococcus salivarius* showed drastic reduction in the formation of clusters of abnormal tubelike glands in the lining of the colon and rectum, as well as a reduction in colonic tumors.

- In a 2012 French study, researchers found that milk fermented with *Propionibacterium freudenreichii* caused cell death, or apoptosis, in human gastric cancer cells. Researchers speculate that long-term use of such milk may prevent the development of gastric cancer, which affects nearly 1 million people each year worldwide.

Eczema and Atopic Dermatitis

Dermatitis is an allergic response, which, some researchers say, indicates digestive abnormalities—specifically compromised gut flora—which has been shown to improve through daily supplement of probiotics, particularly *Lactobacillus GG*.

Epilepsy

Epilepsy is a common neurological disorder among patients with gastrointestinal tract issues. It has been suggested that seizures often result from a damaged gut wall (leaky gut) and from other nutritional deficiencies. Prior to anticonvulsant medications, treatment was only accomplished through dietary supplements and a high-fat diet (called the ketogenic diet). But with the discovery of anticonvulsant drugs in the late 1930s, dietary measures took a backseat. As with all long-term use of chemical medications, they are not without their side effects, and some can damage the mucous lining in the gastrointestinal tract and disrupt the microbial composition.

Seizures place enormous demand on the nutritional status of the body, leaving the person depleted of many essential nutrients. Patients must compensate for such deficiencies as B1, B3, B6, manganese, and folic acid, all of which play a potential role in causing seizures. This is where probiotic-rich fermented foods can be of therapeutic value by repopulating the digestive tract with the beneficial bacteria and helping repair digestive and immune system function. Probiotics can help restore digestive system function and improve absorption of important vitamins, minerals, and essential fatty acids.

Fibromyalgia and Chronic Fatigue Syndrome

Approximately 10 million Americans suffer from fibromyalgia and many more from chronic fatigue syndrome. Both cause debilitating fatigue, but fibromyalgia is characterized by generalized aching, pain, and tenderness throughout the body. Though the exact cause of fibromyalgia is not fully known, there is usually an immune system, digestive system, and nervous system connection.

People with fibromyalgia have nutritional deficiencies and often have digestive system disorders such as IBS, as well as candida yeast infections. This can lead to chronic fatigue, pain, and inflammation throughout the body as well as immune system challenges. Probiotics can reduce these symptoms. When treating chronic fatigue syndrome, it's important to address digestive function, dysbiosis (including candida and parasites), and intestinal flora, as well as to restore immune system function.

Medical histories of people with fibromyalgia often point to triggering events such as a viral or bacterial infection. Often the patient has been prescribed a number of pharmaceuticals ranging from antibiotics to antidepressants, painkillers, and steroids in an effort to address the underlying conditions and accompanying symptoms. All of these medications upset the delicate balance of the microflora and alter the pH in the gut. The patient is then prone to acquiring a variety of inflammatory bowel disorders and intestinal bacterial overgrowth. Malabsorption and vitamin and mineral deficiencies are also prevalent. More research is clearly needed into the therapeutic possibilities of probiotics on these conditions.

Hepatic Encephalopathy (HE)

This brain condition occurs when the liver can no longer detoxify the blood. Certain probiotics, such as *Bifidobacteria*, *Lactobacillus plantarum*, *L. acidophilus*, *L. casei*, and *L. delbrueckii bulgaricus*, have been shown to have superior therapeutic effects compared to conventional treatment that could disrupt the origin of HE and lower the risk of bleeding.

HIV Infection

Human immunodeficiency virus (HIV) is a virus that causes acquired immunodeficiency syndrome (AIDS), a condition that attacks the immune system by destroying important cells that fight disease and infection. This destruction of immune system cells allows life-threatening pathogens and cancers to thrive because the immune system can no longer fight off infections that it would normally be able to prevent.

Since the beginning of the HIV epidemic in 1981, the World Health Organization estimates that more than 60 million people have been infected with HIV worldwide and approximately 30 million people have died of AIDS.

Not surprisingly, nutrient deficiencies and malabsorption are common problems in people with HIV because bacterial overgrowth and dysbiosis can easily occur from the patient's susceptibility to bacterial infections. This can be a result of the disturbance of the microbiota, which appears early in HIV infection and leads to greater dominance of potential pathogens, thereby reducing levels of *Bifidobacteria* and *Lactobacillus* species and increasing mucosal inflammation. HIV patients often have frequent episodes of diarrhea and vomiting along with the malabsorption of important nutrients that are associated with it.

Probiotics have direct enhancement effects on the immune response and defend against invading pathogens. Probiotics can improve the gut's terrain and strengthen both immunity and digestion.

Supporting research conducted at Cornell University in children with HIV infection have shown that administering probiotics has proven effective against infectious diarrhea associated with HIV. According to the four trials Cornell conducted, oral administration of *Lactobacillus plantarum* influenced growth and immune development in children congenitally exposed to HIV who were characterized as having failure to thrive. The immune response may further be enhanced when one or more probiotic strains are consumed together and work synergistically. This seems to be the case when *Lactobacillus* is used in conjunction with *Bifidobacteria*.

In 2003, a study conducted in Tanzania, Africa, sought to assist HIV/AIDS patients by using probiotic yogurt. The probiotic bacteria *Lactobacillus rhamnosus GR-1* was used to make the yogurt, which was created locally in a community kitchen. After beginning to eat yogurt, almost all of the participants gained weight had significantly fewer fungal conditions, had fewer episodes of diarrhea, had greater levels of a number of nutrients, and showed a substantial decrease in fatigue. Overall, this has promising implications for using probiotic-rich fermented foods in treating HIV.

Kidney Stones

Probiotics improve stomach acid production, which helps break down proteins for nutrient absorption, as well as inhibits growth of pathogenic bacteria. Probiotics also correct the body's pH levels by preventing the buildup of uric acid that causes kidney stones.

Obesity

Obesity is a major global health concern. Worldwide, there are more than 1 billion overweight adults, and at least 300 million of them suffer from obesity. It used to be seen primarily in adults over the age of forty-five. Now, it's becoming more common in children who are not just becoming obese, but morbidly obese. Since the early 1980s the prevalence of childhood obesity in America alone has more than tripled among adolescents and teens aged twelve to nineteen, has tripled among youth aged six to eleven, and has more than doubled among children aged two to five.

People who adhere to the standard American diet seem to have the biggest challenges with weight issues. A diet high in sugary, processed carbohydrates, and low in fresh, raw vegetables and fruits not only adds fat and calories to the body but also influences the internal environment of gut flora. Given that the microflora contributes to metabolism—how quickly we burn off calories and convert food into energy—could probiotics offer a solution?

Although the precise cause of obesity is uncertain, we do know that a digestive component and damaged metabolism exists. Most of the obesity studies conducted to date in regard to microflora have focused on animal models, and more research is needed on humans. However, the research provides confirmation that microflora is an important factor in metabolism, obesity, and diabetes.

Evidence shows that our microflora play an important role in breaking down the food we eat, contributing enzymes, and creating nutrients the body can use. In studies conducted at Washington University on human twins, where one twin was obese and one lean, substantial differences were found in the composition of the gut microflora—specifically, in the two dominant groups of beneficial bacteria, the Bacteroidetes and the Firmicutes, which help break down otherwise indigestible foods. The study also showed a decrease in the diversity of microbes that contribute to metabolism, indicating an overall reduction in immunity, in turn creating inflammation. These findings, though preliminary, indicate that obesity has a microbial component, which might have conceivable therapeutic implications.

More research on gut microbiota as a causal factor in the development of obesity and diabetes is clearly needed, but the studies so far are encouraging. Given that the friendly bacteria in fermented foods manufacture important vitamin, and increase protein, mineral, and enzyme content, as well as enhance their bioavailability and assimilation, these friends with benefits also help our body absorb more nutrients, possibly requiring less calories.

Psychiatric Diseases

In the broadest strokes, we can define psychiatric disorders as a psychological pattern of behavior associated with distress that affects how a person thinks, feels, acts, and perceives. In her book *Gut and Psychology Syndrome (GAPS)*, Natasha Campbell-McBride, MD, explains that most psychiatric patients are also dealing with digestive disorders and that there is a link between mental illness symptoms and abnormal gut flora. The gastrointestinal tracts of these patients contain many toxins that are produced by abnormal microflora, which, due to a weakness in the gut wall, are then absorbed into the blood and spread throughout the body.

Schizophrenia is a prime example. It is a complicated disease to diagnose and often overlaps with depression, bipolar disorder, obsessive-compulsive disorder, and dyslexia. Studies have confirmed that people with schizophrenia are often deficient in such vitamins as B1, B3, B6, B12, folic acid, and C, as well as minerals such as magnesium, zinc, and manganese. Successful management of schizophrenic patients with a nutritionally balanced diet, one that avoids gluten and includes vitamins and minerals, has been well documented.

Dr. Campbell-McBride expanded this research further by exploring the gut flora connection to a variety of psychiatric disorders. Her work revealed that when pathogenic microbial flora get the upper hand in the digestive tract, it produces a constant river of toxicity that flows from the gut to the brain. This toxicity is likely behind the symptoms of these disorders in both children and adults.

Toxicity created by the abnormal microflora in the person's gastrointestinal tract could potentially have a negative impact on the brain and lies behind many psychiatric disorder–related symptoms like schizophrenia. As such, it is recommended that treatment be approached from a holistic perspective, including a reduction of the abnormal flora inhabiting the patient and causing toxicity. Dietary and nutritional adjustments are therefore in order.

Sinusitis

Probiotics reduce inflammation and restore immune tolerance toward potential allergens that exacerbate sinus symptoms.

Urogenital Infections

These include bacterial and yeast vaginitis. Probiotics promote activity against pathogenic bacteria species, possibly by producing an acidic environment, and by providing a bacterial barrier able to interfere with the ability of the pathogens to colonize the vagina, and thus reduce the risk of the pathogens ascending into the bladder.

More long-term, well-controlled human studies are critically needed to evaluate the positive preliminary findings of the health benefits of probiotics and the fermented foods that contain them. Considering the known benefits of probiotics, however, it makes sense to regularly consume them for their preventive effects against both acute and chronic diseases.

FERMENTED FOODS TO THE RESCUE

What can we do to inhibit any unfortunate cycle of disease or stave off new diseases from forming? Ideally, we'd make a lifestyle change by adding fermented foods (rather than supplements) to our diet. Lacto-fermented foods are a natural way to stimulate the body to produce its own stomach acid, as opposed to relying solely on a supplement. Consuming lacto-fermented vegetables and fruits will prepare the stomach to properly digest an incoming meal. Once the stomach acid is able to properly digest the food, it will also be able to provoke the pancreas to do its job by secreting its own enzymes as well. Raw foods are a great selection because they provide their own enzymes. They also cleanse and detoxify us. Raw foods can provide much in the way of nourishment, but if we ferment them we can also harness their probiotic qualities.

I've been adding fermented foods to my own and my family's daily diet for a couple of years, and the health benefits and results continue to amaze me. From higher levels of energy, to clearer, younger-looking skin, a healthier digestive system, and stronger immunity, the effects of fermented foods are foundational for building optimal health. Fermented foods undeniably provide a natural method of disease prevention and treatment. Their continued use is essential to maintaining good health. They've been used by civilizations around the world for centuries, and they're now receiving support in establishing their significance in medicine and healing. Think of them as the forgotten superfood that they truly are. In part 2 we'll explore how to make fermented food a natural and enjoyable part of your daily fare and discuss easy ways to transition them into your and your family's lifestyle.

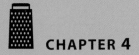

CHAPTER 4

Starting Out with Cultured Food

"Those who think they have not the time for healthy eating and active living will sooner or later have to find time for illness and disease."

— HIPPOCRATES

Preserving foods by fermentation is both an art and a science that has made important contributions to human diets for thousands of years—and continues to do so today. In essence, fermentation is a form of cultivation that helps make the nutrients naturally present in the food more digestible, palatable, and widely available than would be possible without it. Thus, when we ferment foods to make them more nutritious and digestible, we are culturing them—and culturing, by definition, means there's a certain level of sophistication involved.

Generally, the term "culture" is used to define a process of cultivation, or improvements, used in reference to human capacities such as language, social habits, music, arts, and cuisine—human activities that bind people together and can be passed from one generation to the next. But because "culture" is also used to describe foods that are alive with beneficial bacteria, enhanced through the fermentation processes, eating fermented foods can help create a synergy between humans, their societies, and their food. In this chapter, we'll discuss the nutritional qualities of these cultured foods and how you can put this cultural synergy to work for you.

SAFETY OF FERMENTED FOODS

With all the talk of bacteria and pathogens, you may be wondering about the taste of food made with bacteria and whether it's safe to eat. Given society's unfavorable view of bacterial microorganisms and their involvement in the fermentation process, the safety of these foods—be it milk, beans, fish, cabbage, and all manner of foods in between—may surprise you. What makes them safe for consumption? There are several principles at work, most of which we discussed in chapter 1:

Principle #1: Lactic Acid. The proliferation of desirable microorganisms prevents a food from becoming overgrown with unhealthy microbes. Because pathogens are less able to thrive in an acidic environment, the lactic acid by-product of lacto-fermentation helps protect against disease-causing microorganisms by lowering the body's pH.

Principle #2: Alcohol. Alcohol fermentations produce ethanol, which is germicidal; these foods also have longer shelf lives.

Principle #3: Acetic Acid. The production of acetic acid extends preservation even beyond that of ethanol. Depending on the amount, acetic acid can inhibit pathogenic bacteria from reproducing or even kill the bacteria altogether. That is why vinegar is such a common commercial condiment for pickling and preserving vegetables. (It's also why it makes for such a good household cleaner!)

Principle #4: Yeast. When yeast leavens (raises) bread, the carbon dioxide by-product creates an anaerobic environment (without oxygen). When baked, the carbon dioxide leaves a dry surface on the bread that can't be invaded by pathogens. The baking process itself kills microorganisms in the bread, adding to its overall safety.

Principle #5: Mold. Mold fermentations result in antibiotic activity that inhibits putrefying organisms. Molds produce enzymes, and the enzymes act as fermentation catalysts that break down food for the molds to eat.

Principle #6: Alkaline Fermentations. *Bacillus subtilis* are the main microorganisms involved in alkaline fermentation, which breaks down proteins and releases ammonia. This ammonia results in an increased pH, and the high pH and excess ammonia inhibit pathogenic and spoilage microorganisms from invading.

Principle #7: Salt. Adding salt to foods high in protein causes a chemical breakdown that inhibits spoiling and food poisoning, and produces savory sauces and pastes.

In some rare instances, fermented foods can be overtaken by mold or become spoiled. This spoilage can be caused by environmental conditions such as temperature or water levels and is generally not beneficial, because these spoiling organisms can crowd out the beneficial ones. A good rule of thumb in such cases is to throw out the result and start anew.

FERMENTED FOOD ALL-STARS

There are literally hundreds of fermented foods and beverages with origins in cultures the world over; we look at several dozen in this book. However, there are a few all-star players worth getting to know for their immune-boosting probiotic bacteria and nutritional benefits, as well as for their popularity in the traditional foods community.

Yogurt

Made from milk fermented with the lactic acid bacteria *L. acidophilus*, yogurt is the most frequently purchased probiotic food. (*S. thermophilus*, *L. bulgaricus*, and other *Lactobacilli* and *Bifidobacteria* are also sometimes added to improve both taste and digestibility.) However, yogurt can provide greater health benefits if you make it at home, which allows you to control exactly what goes into it, without having to worry about added sugar, chemicals, and pasteurization. Many commercially produced yogurts are subjected to high temperatures during pasteurization, which does not culture or ferment the food but rather destroys beneficial bacteria and enzymes.

It is therefore best to use raw milk, if possible, to retain both its beneficial bacteria and its nutritional value, which will ultimately be enhanced by fermenting it. A probiotic yogurt sold at the store may only have been fermented for a relatively short time and will not have reached its full capacity of beneficial gut flora. The longer the fermentation, the less lactose remains; after twenty-four hours, no lactose remains, which is ideal for those with lactose intolerance.

Yogurt is high in protein, calcium, riboflavin, and B vitamins. The probiotics present in yogurt have been found successful in treating diarrhea caused by antibiotics, because they are able to replace some of the good bacteria in the gastrointestinal tract that are often unintentionally destroyed by the antibiotic.

A Test for Live Yogurt

Some yogurt products claim to contain "live" bacteria, which you can easily test for at home. Mix 1 tablespoon (15 g) of the live yogurt with 1 cup (235 ml) of heated (but not boiled) milk and leave it in a warm place overnight. If the mixture has thickened by morning, there are live cultures present.

Kefir

Originating in northern Russia in the early 1900s, kefir is a milk product made from kefir grains, which are composed of colonies of live *Lactobacillus* bacteria and yeasts bound together in a symbiotic relationship and fermented at room temperature. Kefir is created in a similar process to yogurt and has a similar tart flavor and creamy consistency. It is more healthful than its commercial counterpart because of its beneficial bacteria. These microorganisms predigest the kefir, enhancing it with vitamins and minerals, which then require less effort for our digestive tract to metabolize. They also digest lactose in milk during fermentation, because milk contains the enzyme lactase, making kefir ideal for those who are lactose intolerant.

Kefir even possesses natural antibiotics. It is rich in vitamins B1 and B12, calcium, folic acid, phosphorus, and vitamin K. Some people instantly take to kefir, while others may need to introduce it into the diet in small amounts (a teaspoon at first) until their bodies build up a tolerance through regular consumption. Although it's simple to make at home, kefir is now widely available at health food stores and many supermarkets.

Sauerkraut

Sauerkraut is one of the oldest fermented foods and today is eaten mostly in Germany, Russia, and Eastern Europe. It can be made with white or red cabbage, and traditionally only has salt added. (see page 93 for a recipe). Originally discovered as a healthful therapeutic aid for the digestive tract, sauerkraut is still used for its digestive enzymes, probiotic bacteria, lactic acid, vitamins, and minerals. It is often eaten with meats to aid in their digestion by providing its own enzymes to help break down the meat and to engage stomach acid. Even fresh cabbage will naturally ferment without adding fermenting bacteria to it because it contains its own healthy bacteria. These healthy bacteria eat the cabbage and give off lactic acid, which in turn makes the sauerkraut sour and kills pathogenic bacteria.

The lactic acid is what can preserve unpasteurized sauerkraut for more than a year in the refrigerator. The key word here is "unpasteurized." The commercial pasteurization of kraut stabilizes it so it can be sold in stores without needing refrigeration; unfortunately, at the same time, it detracts from the food's health benefits because the heat destroys its natural enzymes and healthy bacteria. You must ask for unpasteurized sauerkraut if you wish to receive its health benefits! Like many commercially produced dairy products, most commercially produced sauerkraut, pickles, and other plant foods have been processed only with vinegar as a base and have been subjected to high temperatures, which does not culture or ferment the food.

The preventive health measures and preservative abilities of the lactic acid in sauerkraut perform the same functions in the large intestine. Eating sauerkraut will boost your immune system through its high vitamin C content and provides cancer-fighting antioxidants. Sauerkraut also contains large quantities of acetylcholine, which helps lower blood pressure and slows heartbeat, thus promoting a sense of calmness important for restful sleep. It has also shown beneficial effects on peristalsis, which ensures gastric emptying and regular bowel movements. Introduce this extraordinary food into your diet slowly to allow your gastrointestinal tract to get used to its cleansing effects. Eat it in small quantities (even just a single bite) regularly, and ten to fifteen minutes before a meal if you have low stomach acidity, to aid in digestion.

Kimchi

Kimchi is another form of cabbage that undergoes lacto-fermentation and can take up to a year to ferment fully, depending on how strong a taste you like. It is the national dish of Korea and dates back to the seventh century. The average Korean eats around 40 pounds (18 kg) of kimchi every year, and kimchi is believed to have helped keep obesity rates lower in Korea than other countries because of its low calorie count. Depending on the region and what's in season, Koreans sometimes use other vegetables, such as cucumbers and scallions, and combine them with chile, garlic, onions, and ginger. Kimchi (see page 100 for a recipe) possesses anticarcinogenic effects and is packed with vitamin A, thiamin, riboflavin, calcium, and iron. It's well known for its tangy, spicy, acidic taste and is eaten for breakfast, lunch, and dinner in Korea.

Miso

Miso is a traditional Chinese paste from the third century BCE that is commonly used as a seasoning and in soups. To make miso, soybeans are soaked, cooked, mashed, and hung to ferment for about a month until they have been completely overgrown with *Aspergillus oryzae* mold. It is then placed in salt brine, covered with a lid, and allowed to sit undisturbed under moderate temperature, which allows the fermenting process to begin and produces an amino acid–rich paste with a savory and salty flavor. (Generally, the longer it's been aged, the darker the color—from yellow to red to deep brown—and the stronger and saltier the taste.) Miso contributes essential amino acids and other nutrients such as extensive probiotics, vitamin B12, and antioxidants to the foods it flavors. Various studies have suggested that these nutrients help protect against radiation, breast cancer, and pathogen infection.

Tempeh

Tempeh is a two-thousand-year-old Indonesian fermented food that's often used in place of meat. Made by culturing partially cooked soybeans with *Rhizopus oligosporus* mold, the soybeans are soaked for thirty-six to forty-eight hours in the starter mold, which results in an acidic pH that inhibits many detrimental organisms but is fine for the mold. This produces a somewhat nutty flavor and a texture similar to a chewy mushroom as it goes through the fermentation process. Then the surface is dried, inhibiting putrefying bacterial growth. The mold proliferates rapidly at high temperatures that other pathogenic bacteria and mold could not thrive in. The mold also produces natural, heat-stable antibiotic agents against some disease-causing organisms.

Unlike other fermented foods, however, tempeh must be cooked, which rids it of more undesirable microorganisms. And unlike other plant foods, fermented soybeans in tempeh contain vitamin B12, a by-product of the fermentation process. This is important, especially for vegans and vegetarians who are often deficient in B12, which can lead to anemia and irreversible nerve damage. B12 is also a necessary vitamin for pregnant and lactating women.

Although it seems similar to tofu (a soft cheese-like food made by curdling soy milk), tempeh provides greater nutritional value because it contains whey and is predigested by its own natural bacteria, thereby enhancing the body's absorption of the isoflavones found in soy that provide health-protective functions. The fermentation process also removes the counterproductive enzymeinhibitors that occur naturally in soybeans. These inhibitors interfere with protein digestion and block the enzyme's healthful activity inside your body (such as improving digestion). All legumes, grains, and seeds contain enzymeinhibitors, which are kept dormant until they are soaked or fermented. Soaking and fermenting all legumes, grains, and seeds releases all of their nutrients so that they are more usable and digestible in your intestines.

Tempeh is high in fiber, enzymes, manganese, and beneficial bacteria and is a good digestible protein source—and it's a great meat substitute that is high in protein. It is an excellent source of calcium and plant protein, containing all of the essential amino acids. It is not easily produced at home, but it is readily available in most health food stores and some major supermarkets. Because many soybean crops are genetically modified, it is best to purchase only organic brands. Even though most traditional tempeh is made from soybeans, sometimes you will find that it contains a blend of grains, beans, or other vegetables and is just as healthful and tasty. Either way, similarly to tofu, it tends to absorb the flavors of the other ingredients cooked along with it.

Natto

Natto is a traditional Japanese food made from soybeans sprinkled with *Bacillus subtilis* bacteria and soaked for twenty-four hours. It dates back to over a thousand years ago, when it became a popular Japanese staple. It has a strong, nutty, salty flavor, and a pungent odor. Often considered an acquired taste for most Westerners, it is celebrated as a delicacy in Japan, where it is mostly eaten at breakfast with rice, miso, hot mustards, raw egg, and assorted vegetables. It is available at selected markets and online suppliers in the United States. Typically, natto soybeans are used because these are smaller than regular soybeans, allowing the fermentation process to more easily reach the center of the bean.

Nutritionally, natto has a lot to offer. It is a rich source of protein, containing as much as in a similar amount of beef. It is high in vitamins K, B2, and E, as well as antioxidants, particularly selenium. Natto also contains an enzyme called nattokinase, which is produced during the fermentation process. Nattokinase has been shown to have anti-inflammatory health benefits and to be helpful in preventing and treating blood clots. It works by breaking down fibrin, a protein that in excess can contribute to heart disease, stroke, poor circulation, and slow tissue repair.

The Discovery of the Blood-Clot-Busting Effects of Nattokinase

In 1980, medical doctor and researcher Hiroyuki Suma, MD, who was majoring in physiological chemistry at the University of Chicago, accidentally discovered nattokinase. Dr. Suma was searching for a natural agent that could successfully dissolve blood clots (known as thrombus) that form in a blood vessel and cause heart attacks and strokes. He dropped a small portion of the natto he was eating for lunch into the artificial thrombus (called fibrin, a protein involved in the clotting of blood) in a Petri dish. Within eighteen hours, the natto had completely dissolved the thrombus and showed a potency unmatched by any other enzyme. He named the fribrinolytic enzyme "nattokinase."

Kombucha

Hailed as an elixir of life, kombucha (see chapter 12) is a fermented mushroom tea relied on both as a medicinal beverage and as a generally healthful concoction. The first recorded use of kombucha comes from China in 221 BCE, where it was called "Immortal Health Elixir." It is filled with enzymes and amino acids that inhibit pathogenic activity while fortifying the gastrointestinal tract. It destroys toxins found in the body using glucaric acetate, a process that also helps engage the stomach during digestion and aids the absorption of key nutrients. It also provides antioxidants and helps maintain the pH in the body, both of which contribute to its positive effect on our immune system.

Kombucha is available commercially at selected markets and health food stores, and of course you can make it at home yourself using a kombucha culture, which is often referred to as the "mushroom" or the "mother." The fermentation process of this beverage produces up to 1.5 percent ethyl alcohol content, with increased brewing time increasing the percentage of alcohol. For those who do not wish to consume alcoholic beverages, rejuvelac is a great alternative.

Rejuvelac

Rejuvelac, promoted by world-renowned naturopath and raw food expert Ann Wigmore, ND, of the Natural Health Institute in Aguada, Puerto Rico, is a probiotic drink made of sprouts grown from such grains as wheat berries, rye, and quinoa. Other ingredients such as barley, oats, and buckwheat may also be used to make rejuvelac. It has a slightly sour, lemony taste, and is most refreshing (see page 182 for a recipe).

Used to improve digestion by adding beneficial enzymes and bacteria to the gastrointestinal tract, it is rejuvenating, hence its name. The bacteria added to our digestive system by drinking this beverage help clean our gastrointestinal tract and remove toxins and other wastes. Rejuvelac is high in amino acids—the building blocks of protein—that have been broken down into an easy to assimilate form. For people who have problems breaking down their proteins—perhaps as a result of disorders such as gluten intolerance, Crohn's disease, or low levels of hydrochloric acid in the stomach—rejuvelac may provide aid. Rejuvelac is rich in *Lactobacillus* and the mold *Aspergillus oryzae* that converts starches into sugar, and contains vitamins C, E, and eight of the B-complex vitamins that aid the central nervous system and fight stress. Rejuvelac is excellent for blending into seed and nut milks, or sauces, and for making seed yogurt and cheese because its high vitamin E content is an anti-oxidant that stops fats from oxidizing.

NOURISHING OURSELVES BY CULTIVATING OUR MICROFLORA

The amount of nutrients available in the average adult diet has declined over the past few decades as we have moved further away from our traditional food roots. Fortunately, we have the power to change this by selecting from a variety of healthful, fresh foods that nourish our bodies with essential vitamins, minerals, protein, carbohydrates, fats, and enzymes. It's important that you select healthful foods from five basic food groups to get the nutrients your body needs. When you start with a core of healthful food groups—dairy, grains and legumes, vegetables and fruits, meats and fish, and healthful fats—fermentation simply amplifies the best these foods have to offer. We'll walk through each of them and discuss how to work within their range of offerings to increase consumption of prebiotics and probiotics in your diet.

Dairy Products

Lacto-fermented dairy products are naturally higher in probiotics—primarily *Lactobacillus acidophilus*, *Lactobacillus casei*, and *Bifidobacteria*—and contain more vitamins and minerals compared to non-fermented dairy. Enjoyed for centuries, they have been used mainly as a protective and preventive measure against disease rather than as a therapeutic one. Milk and dairy products provide an excellent carrier for these probiotic organisms because most of them can readily use lactose (milk sugar) as an energy source for growth. Milk proteins also protect the probiotic bacteria while they pass through the stomach. The potential health benefits from consuming lacto-fermented dairy products containing probiotic, include the following:

- enhanced stimulation or modulation of the immune system
- improved levels of serum cholesterol
- improved use of lactose and other nutrients
- better control of intestinal infections
- reduced risk of certain cancers

The best sources of fermented dairy are yogurt and kefir and some aged cheeses that contain live probiotic bacteria. Enjoy them on a daily basis.

Grains and Beans

Cereal grains have long been considered one of the most important groups of food crops and are a staple in many cultures worldwide. Cereal grains are the fruit of plants belonging to the grass family, which includes wheat, barley, rice, maize, millet, rye, sorghum, oats, kamut, spelt, and triticale. Nutritionally, they are valuable sources of dietary protein, carbohydrates, fiber, B-complex vitamins, vitamin E, iron, and trace minerals selenium, copper, manganese, and zinc. They are more energy dense than most vegetables and fruits, meaning they contain more calories, so you don't need to eat a lot to feel full. The nutritional value of cereal grains and their products (most notably flour and breakfast cereals) is substantially reduced during the refining and milling process, which is why they are often enriched after processing. But the ratio and amounts of nutrients put back after refining are different than what the plant naturally contains, making them somewhat inferior in nutritional value and content.

Most cereal grains contain a certain amount of secondary metabolites, which are compounds that are not essential for the growth or survival of the grain and tend to be either toxic or anti-nutritional to us. Phytates, enzyme inhibitors, protease (protein) inhibitors, tannins, saponins, lectins, and gluten can all be toxicants and anti-nutrients in the human body to some extent.

Replacing refined grains with whole grains that have the whole grain intact (ones that contain the bran, germ, and endosperm) and are not genetically modified is by far the most wholesome choice. Selecting these will ensure that you are getting the vitamins, minerals, fiber, and other health factors that you lose with refined grains. Soaking and sprouting them in nonchlorinated water for at least twenty-four hours prior to cooking or heating releases the enzyme inhibitors, decreases phytates and other toxicants, and makes protein and other nutrients more available for your body to digest. Fermenting the soaked or sprouted grains allows beneficial bacteria and enzymes to work their magic by further breaking down complex starches, tremendously increasing their nutritional value.

Together with grains, beans and other legumes supply a majority of dietary protein, complex carbohydrates, fiber, vitamins, and minerals necessary in the human diet. Beans, lentils, and peas have been shown to provide many health benefits including:

- lowering cholesterol, triglycerides, and blood pressure

- keeping blood sugar levels stable

- lowering risk for certain types of cancers, particularly colon and breast cancer

- reducing inflammation in the body

- reducing risk of coronary artery disease, diabetes, and osteoporosis

But their health benefits do not stop there. Among all food groups commonly eaten worldwide, no group has a more health-supportive mix of protein plus fiber than beans. With 40 grams of protein per cup (equivalent to 4 ounces [113 g] of meat), they are a perfect food for vegetarians and vegans. Further, a single, 1-cup (62-g) serving of black beans, for example, provides nearly 15 grams of fiber, which is well over half the recommended daily value in the United States. In addition to satisfying your appetite, the high fiber content in beans aids in digestion and weight loss. Foods that are rich in both protein and fiber (which only beans are) promote greater movement of food through the gastrointestinal tract, allowing gastric emptying to occur at a more desirable pace. This greater efficiency supports both optimal balance of nutrients and growth of beneficial microorganisms. Up to 40 percent of the starch, fiber, and protein in beans is actually unavailable to us for digestion in the small intestine and is moved through to the large intestine, where it serves to provide the perfect mix of substances for encouraging friendly bacterial growth. This indigestible portion of a food is called the dietary indigestible fraction (DIF). The DIF values of certain beans—especially black beans, chickpeas, and lentils—have been shown to act as prebiotic substances that allow bacteria in the colon to produce butyric acid. The cells lining the inside of the colon can use this butyric acid to fuel their many immune-enhancing activities and keep the lower digestive tract functioning properly.

Beans are high in enzyme inhibitors as well as phytates, which we know are highly indigestible and block the absorption of the important minerals calcium, magnesium, iron, and zinc, and, ironically enough, reduce the absorption of protein. Simply cooking the beans or sprouting them is not sufficient to break down the phytic acid they contain. Rinsing and then soaking your beans overnight in very warm water (140°F [60°C]) in a warm space in your kitchen has proven to be a much more effective way to break down the phytates. As the beans absorb water, simply add more warm water to keep them moist. However, the most effective method to reduce the phytates and increase the nutritional benefits of beans is to ferment them. Be sure to purchase beans that have not been genetically modified (GMO free) to ensure highest quality and safety.

Vegetables and Fruits

Fruits and vegetables provide an abundant supply of fiber and other health-supportive compounds that encourage the growth of probiotics. Among these compounds are antioxidants, which protect the cells in your body from free radical damage and play a significant role in preventing degenerative disease.

There are three major groups of antioxidants: carotenoids (related to vitamin A), allyl sulfides (found in garlic and onions), and the largest group, the polyphenols (common constituents of foods of plant origin). Several hundred different types of polyphenols have been identified in foods, of which the two main types are flavonoids and phenolic acids. (Of the total intake of polyphenols in our diet, flavonoids account for two-thirds and phenolic acids account for about one-third.) Flavonoids are themselves distributed among several classes: flavones, flavonols, flavanones, isoflavones, proanthocyanidins, and anthocyanins. Here are some of the most common flavonoids:

- quercetin, a flavonol abundant in apples, onions, broccoli, and green tea
- anthocyanins, found in a large number of fruits and vegetables (particularly grapes, berries, and grapeseed extract) and which give brilliant color to many red fruits (raspberry, strawberry, and blackberry)

- proanthocyanidins, common in many fruits and responsible for their characteristic astringency or bitterness
- catechins, a flavonol found in tea and several fruits, such as berries and apples
- hesperidin, a flavanone present in citrus fruits
- isoflavones, which include genistein and daidzein found in soy

Phenolic acids are simple molecules such as caffeic acid (present in many fruits and vegetables and in coffee), vanillin (from processed vanilla bean), and courmaric acid (present in grapes and wine).

Polyphenols are linked to cancer prevention, antitumor growth, anti-inflammatory properties, cardiovascular support, and protection against harmful pathogens. Apart from the many health benefits and prebiotic effects that these naturally occurring polyphenols bestow upon us, it turns out that these compounds are picked up and used by the beneficial bacteria in the digestive system. Studies show that the health effects of polyphenols depend on their intake and bioavailability, and that eating plant products on a daily basis is necessary to maintain high concentrations of the organic compounds of polyphenols in the blood. Fermented foods such as cabbage, carrots, asparagus, soybeans, capers, olives, plums, berries, and other vegetables and fruits contain a wide range of beneficial polyphenols.

Meat and Fish

Meat and fish both contain all of the essential and nonessential amino acids the body needs to produce protein. While vegetables, grains, and beans contain amino acids, they do not contain the full complement of amino acids the body needs to formulate a complete protein. You would have to combine them with another plant-based food that contains amino acids—such as pairing beans with rice—so together they form a complete protein.)

● Advice for Choosing Raw Meat and Fish For Fermenting

Folks have been fermenting meats and fish pretty much since the start of civilization. The biggest consideration for most people today when they ferment meats and fish is ensuring the growth of pathogenic organisms. Therefore, you will want to select raw meat that is fresh and of highest quality. Choose meat from an animal that has been raised without the use of antibiotics, which can prevent growth of friendly microorganisms, and preferably grown in optimum environments, such as organically. Wild-caught fish is superior to farm raised because they will have a minimal bacterial load and are free of antibiotics. Meat should be well trimmed, free of connective tissue, glands, and blood clots. Lean meats contain moisture and will ferment faster. The color of lean fat is also important: intense red lean is preferable to yellow fat, which should be avoided. Be sure to use water that is not chlorinated, as this can retard growth of beneficial microorganisms, and remember to rinse your meat and fish well before fermenting it. Feel free to add herbs and spices to your meats and fish to enhance their flavors.

Meats such as beef, veal, pork, lamb, chicken, turkey, and duck are high in the essential B-complex vitamins, along with vitamins E, D, and K. They also contain high amounts of necessary minerals, such as potassium, magnesium, calcium, phosphorus, zinc, iron, copper, and selenium. The meat from animals that have been grass-fed and are organic is the best choice. Commercially grown cattle receive antibiotics and other chemicals that inevitably end up in the muscles and organs of these animals and are then passed on to you.

Fish is an excellent source of omega-3 essential fatty acids, an essential nutrient our body cannot make. Omega-3s are necessary for such bodily processes as building cell membranes in the brain and improving brain function, increasing HDL (good) cholesterol, lowering triglycerides and the risk of heart disease, reducing inflammation in the body, eliminating joint pain, and easing depression, and they act as anticoagulants to prevent blood from clotting. The best sources are from coldwater deep sea fish such as salmon, tuna, sardines, mackerel, herring, trout, and halibut. To avoid or minimize mercury intake, choose fish that are lower on the food chain (such as sardines and herring) or that have been found to be low in mercury.

Fermentation not only improves the taste of meat and fish but also makes them easier to digest. Marinating meats and fish before cooking enhances the bioavailability of the vitamin and mineral content and predigests them.

Healthful Fats and Oils

Since the 1920s, we've known that fats are essential in our diets. Dietary fats are required as a major source of fuel for the body. The body needs fat for energy, and tissue repair, and to transport fat-soluble vitamins A, D, E, and K around the body. Beneficial bacteria in fermented foods improve synthesis of essential fatty acids, particularly omega-3s.

The key to making fat work for you is to consume natural fats in balanced amounts. There are two important considerations: The first is to consume a variety of healthful fats from omega-3 and omega-6 sources. These include unrefined oils such as extra-virgin olive oil, coconut oil, sesame oil, flaxseed oil, and grapeseed oil. Fats from butter, ghee, eggs, meats, fish, and dairy are good as well because they are part of a balanced diet. The second is to avoid hydrogenated (or partially hydrogenated) fats and highly processed vegetable oils. These include fats that are solid at room temperature, such as margarine, and many of the fats used to make baked goods, such as vegetable shortening, palm oil, and soybean oil (read labels). Hydrogenated fats (trans fats) disturb the metabolism of fats in the body and lead to chronic diseases such as atherosclerosis, heart disease, and cancer. Fried or cooked fats should also be avoided for similar reasons.

For years we've been steered toward low-fat diets and told by public health officials that diets containing high amounts of animal and saturated fats can raise cholesterol to unhealthy levels and increase the risk for cardiovascular disease and cancer. It's a message that's been all too readily reinforced by the food industry selling us low-fat products and highly processed oils. Several studies, however, have proven conclusively that low-fat diets neither lower cholesterol or reduce the risk for cardiovascular disease and cancer.

Probably the most well known is the Framingham Heart Study, a longevity study that was launched in the 1940s by the National Heart Institute (now known as the National Heart, Lung, and Blood Institute) and that involved fifty-two hundred men and women. It looked at how diet related to cholesterol levels and the development of heart disease. The study showed that cholesterol levels were not associated with an increased risk of heart disease and, in fact, after age forty-seven, those whose cholesterol levels went down had the highest risk of a heart attack. The ongoing Harvard University Nurses' Health Study involving about ninety thousand nurses studied since 1976 shows similar data. An interim report published in 1997 noted that total fat intake, animal fat intake, saturated fat intake, and cholesterol intake were not associated with coronary heart disease.

Fermentation produces short-chain fatty acids (a subgroup of fatty acids, known as SCFAs), and depending on the amounts of microflora present in the colon, these can be readily absorbed and provide a number of health benefits to us. A 2006 Canadian study on the effects of SCFAs produced from fermentation showed that they can improve cholesterol synthesis and may reduce blood fat levels, possibly reducing the risk of cardiovascular disease. The SCFA butyrate was shown to provide nourishment in the colon mucosa, thereby creating a protective effect that may aid in the prevention of cancer of the colon. More studies are needed on the patterns of SCFAs from fermentation, but in the interim, you can easily, and safely, incorporate probiotics through fermented foods into your diet and see some positive changes.

PANTRY STOCKING

It's a lot easier to prepare healthful fermented meals and snacks if you have all the ingredients you need at your fingertips. When your pantry is stocked with healthful staples, you naturally make smarter choices. It doesn't take much to achieve, and there are a few simple guidelines that can make all the difference between ordinary and extraordinary results.

What to Have on Hand to Start Fermenting

If you're planning on making your own fermented foods, you'll want to keep some of these key ingredients handy:
- *a good supply of fresh, clean spring water*
- *sea salt (avoid table salt or iodized salt)*
- *starter cultures, such as whey for making yogurt, dried sourdough starter, kefir grains, a kombucha SCOBY*
- *tempeh (can be kept in the fridge for several weeks or frozen)*
- *coconut milk*
- *whole wheat, spelt, or other flour*
- *vinegar (I like organic apple cider the best.)*
- *a selection of grains and seeds*
- *a jar of sauerkraut (You can never have enough of this!)*

Buy Fresh, Buy Local

Foods grown locally in your own community are the freshest and most nutritious choices, which also means they're better tasting. These qualities are lost in food trucked or flown in from thousands of miles away, plus there is less chance of contamination or irradiation when you buy locally. Fresh foods that are GMO free and organically grown are superior choices for your fermentations. Foods raised with pesticides, fungicides, hormones, and antibiotics are lower in nutrient content, lose vitality, and are less appealing for friendly microorganisms to populate and thrive.

If you look for local farmers who follow organic and sustainable growing practices, you'll avoid genetically modified foods and exposure to pesticides and other harmful chemicals. Knowing your local farmer and where your food comes from also develops a meaningful connection to your food, plus it builds relationships based on trust and understanding within your community. Eating locally grown foods makes it possible for farmers to continue to provide you and your family with a plentiful selection of nutritious foods that will continue to be available for future generations.

Ingredients to Avoid

There are several ingredients that will benefit your fermented food preparations and your health greatly—when you avoid them.

Monosodium glutamate (MSG), which contains the toxic amino acid glutamic acid, is a food additive and flavor enhancer that's added to virtually all processed foods, including ultra-pasteurized milk (and anything made with low-fat, skim, or nonfat milk), and is even sprayed on crops as a growth enhancer. Many serious allergic reactions have been reported following ingestion of produce (particularly lettuce, strawberries, grapes, tomatoes, onions, and russet potatoes) sprayed with a product containing MSG. There are more than ninety-two documented symptoms from ingesting this nerve toxin, including migraine headaches, cardiac arrhythmias, numbness or paralysis, seizures, depression, insomnia, asthma, loss of balance, mental confusion, anxiety, hyperactivity, and behavioral changes in children. This is another good reason to purchase organic produce or those grown locally from reputable sources.

Aspartic acid is another amino acid, found in the sugar substitute aspartame and sold in the United States under the brand names NutraSweet and Equal. Aspartic acids are naturally present in some of the foods we eat, such as seafood, chicken, beef, lamb, soybeans, dairy, and some fruits and vegetables; they're safe when eaten as natural foods that contain other amino acids. Taken alone, however, and in elevated quantities, they are quite toxic and can cause permanent damage to brain cells and the nervous system.

Genetically modified organisms (GMOs) are plants or animals that have been genetically engineered to create a set of "desirable" traits that include increased crop size and yield, extended shelf life, and vibrant color. However, GMOs come at a cost to your health because they are lower in nutrient density, contain toxins, and are hazardous to the environment. There are no longevity studies done on GMO safety because they have not been around long enough. Several short-term studies, however, have shown GMOs to be carcinogenic (cancer-causing), to disrupt the immune system, to contribute to food allergies, and to create super strains of viruses resistant to the chemicals used to create GMOs. Always purchase foods that have not been genetically modified in any way.

Equipment Necessary for Fermentation

If you're planning to create probiotic-rich, lacto-fermented foods at home, you do need a few basic tools and equipment to ensure consistent and predictable results.

Although it's not necessary to purchase expensive equipment, you do want to make sure that your fermenting vessels are made from the right materials, usually ceramic or glass. You'll need a ceramic crock and several wide-mouth glass canning jars, ranging in size from pint to gallon, depending on your needs. (I recommend having a variety of sizes of glass canning jars on hand so you can preserve and store your fermented dishes and to allow you to make a variety of different foods at any given time.) It's best to avoid aluminum, tin, cast iron, or copper containers because these metals can be corrosive and will react with the acids in fermenting foods and inhibit the fermentation process. Plastic is also not recommended because it, too, can leach chemicals and harbor harmful bacteria that can spoil your fermentations. If you do use plastic, perhaps as a food storage container, then be sure to choose food-grade plastic (preferably BPA free) and use it only for food purposes and not to hold other non-food substances.

For some recipes, you'll need a weight to keep your vegetables submerged and to prevent them from floating above the liquid brine (which lends itself to mold forming). This can be done by simply placing a plate that fits snugly inside the vessel, then putting a clean rock, a resealable plastic bag filled with water, or a similar weight on top of the plate to hold down the vegetables. You will also need a covering lid for your glass canning jars or crock to keep bugs out but still allows the gases that are created during fermentation to escape. Keep in mind that lactic acid bacteria thrive in an anaerobic (without oxygen) environment and are neutralized when oxygen is present. When preserving in jars there should always be ½ inch (13 mm) of brine on top of all fermenting vegetables because some liquid will naturally escape the jar as gas. Remember to always store your sealed fermentation jars on a towel for hygienic purposes because sometimes escaping liquid will dribble down the sides and attract competing bacteria.

It's not necessary to spend a lot of money on your fermentation vessels, especially when you are just starting out. However, as you become more experienced and your fermentation finesse expands, you may wish to purchase ceramic crocks or glass jars equipped with weights and airlocks. These are designed to allow the natural gases to escape while sealing out oxygen, thereby reducing or eliminating the threat of mold during the fermentation process. No matter which containers you use, it's important that they are kept squeaky clean. Wash them by hand using hot, soapy water and let them dry in the sun or air-dry naturally— avoid using cloths or towels because these may harbor pathogenic bacteria that could impede your fermentation efforts.

Other useful tools you will need on hand include a cutting board, a vegetable knife, a mandoline slicer or a food processor, and a blunt meat pounder or potato masher to pound juices out of vegetables. Chances are, you probably already have these items in your kitchen.

By eating a variety of fermented food, we promote the growth of an abundant supply of the beneficial helpers that keep us healthy and rejuvenated. As an added benefit, fermentation allow us to eat fresh, locally grown vegetables, rich in enzymes, fiber, vitamins, and minerals, all year-round. Getting used to such foods made more healthful through fermentation helps us strengthen our natural instincts for more healthful eating. It's time to reacquaint ourselves with this centuries-old technique and the exciting world of fermentation.

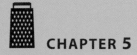

CHAPTER 5

Changing the Way We Eat

"The food you eat can be either the safest and most powerful form of medicine, or the slowest form of poison."

— ANN WIGMORE, ND

When it comes to which foods we put into our bodies, the best choices are the ones that provide the most nourishment. But in our modern world we've become masters of industrial food processing. Natural, whole, indigenous foods have been replaced by refined flour and sugar, soft drinks, and candy bars. Methods such as industrialized canning, freezing, pasteurization, and genetic engineering have taken precedence and become accepted as a normal way of producing food to feed our families.

The safer, more effective and convenient methods to preserve nutrients in food, such as culturing and fermentation, are often judged as strange. And with the increase of commercial production so, too, have we witnessed an increase in chronic degenerative disorders and an emergence of new diseases, some of which weren't even known or heard of before the previous century: HIV/AIDS, metabolic syndrome (also known as syndrome X or insulin resistance syndrome), Lyme disease, T cell leukemia, mad cow (bovine encephalopathy), Morgellans disease, swine flu, peptic ulcer disease (*Helicobacter pylori*), Severe Acute Respritory Syndrome (SARS), hepatitis C and E, cryptosporidiosis, roseola infantum, and toxic shock syndrome. All of these disorders have a nutritional component to them.

Changing the way you eat, however, can be a daunting, even overwhelming task. Fortunately, there is a natural-foods resurgence taking place, and many people are moving toward healthier, more sustainable lifestyles. Traditional fermented foods offer many solutions because they are a naturally rich source of vital nutrients, are energy efficient, and offer a cost-effective means of obtaining desirable results.

In this chapter we will discuss how you can make the positive switch to include fermented foods as a natural part of your daily fare and how you can lay the foundation to optimize health benefits. It doesn't take much effort to make the switch, and there are simple and easy steps you can take that yield countless rewards. It's a lot easier than you might have imagined.

CHOOSING THE RIGHT FOODS

But where do we start, and how do we go about making the best fermented food choices and incorporating them as part of a healthful daily diet? The answer to this question lies in whether you intend to ferment your own foods or want to purchase already fermented foods. Even if you decide to ferment your own foods, I recommend you keep a variety of store-bought fermented foods in your pantry to ensure you always have something healthful to eat at the ready.

With either choice, you will want to maximize the many health benefits by incorporating into your daily diet a variety of fresh, seasonal, whole foods because these contain enzymes that complement fermented foods nicely. This may mean letting go of canned, frozen, pasteurized, or other processed foods that have added chemicals that upset intestinal flora. If cutting out commercially processed foods is difficult, simply add more fresh foods as close to their natural state and season as possible.

There's no shortage of choices when it comes to which foods can be fermented becauase practically every food group offers options.

Use your imagination to come up with combinations and flavors that will delight you, and enjoy these on a daily basis. Always choose the freshest ingredients for fermenting because these will contribute the highest return in terms of their enzymes, minerals, and essential nutrients—not to mention flavor.

Foods That Can Be Fermented	
Food Group	**Fermenting Options**
Vegetables	sauerkraut, pickles, relishes, vinegar, root beer, salsas
Fruits	chutneys, jams, sauces, honey, wines, ciders
Beans	miso, soy sauce, shoyu, natto, tempeh, bean pastes
Grains	sourdough, breads, crackers, muffins
Nuts and seeds	nondairy "cheeses," seed pastes
Dairy	yogurt, buttermilk, sour cream, kefir, crème fraîche, aged cheeses
Fish	fish sauces and pastes
Meat (pork and beef)	sausages, salami, corned beef
Eggs	pickled eggs (can also be used to make mayonnaise)

🥘 Guidelines for Quick Home Fermentation

- *Choose organic produce because they supply more nutrients, especially trace minerals, which must be present in sufficient amounts for enzymes to function.*

- *Wash—but don't scrub—the surface of fruits and vegetables you intend to ferment, and don't use chemicals or detergents to "decontaminate" them because this can inhibit growth of beneficial bacteria.*

- *The more thinly cut your fruits and vegetables, the more surface area for the bacteria to inhabit.*

- *Pack as many vegetables or fruits into your fermenting jar as you can, and cover them with the brine to within ½ inch (13 mm) of the top.*

- *Always use pure, unprocessed sea salt. Remember that the more salt you use, the slower the fermentation will take place—and the more acidic the result will be. If you're using whey as your fermentation starter, then you can use less or even no salt. (Whey also accelerates the fermentation process over brine.)*

- *Most fermented dishes require between ¼ to 1 cup (60–230 ml) of whey.*

- *During the lacto-fermentation process, screw the lid on the jar, leaving it loose enough for the gases that will bubble up inside to escape.*

- *Keep active fermentation jars at room temperature (around 72°F [22°C] is ideal). Above 72°F (22°C) speeds the process, whereas below slows it down.*

- *Do not open or unscrew jars for 3 days to keep oxygen out during this first part of the fermentation process. After 3 days, you can check daily and do a taste test until the vegetables or fruits taste pickled. (They will get softer the longer the fermentation process goes on.)*

- *Transfer finished jars to the refrigerator for storage, which will slow the fermentation process considerably.*

TIPS FOR GETTING STARTED

When making your own lacto-fermented foods, several basic ingredients are required for the process to be effective. Fermentation is simple and easy to do once you have them. Salt, water, and a starter culture are the three main ingredients you need. The salt and water, when combined, make what is called a brine. A starter culture is a set of living beneficial organisms in wet or dry form that gives the food an active colony of microorganisms to start the process of fermentation. This starter culture (usually whey) is the microbiological culture that actually performs the fermentation, and it consists of a cultivation medium, such as grains, seeds, or nutrient liquids that have been well colonized by the microorganisms (bacterial and fungal). Most starter cultures come from *Lactobacillus acidophilus* and *Bifidobacteria* in small quantities of whey retained from previous successful batches of a fermented product. You may need to purchase a starter culture to begin the process (see Resources).

The Why of Whey

Whey is the thin, watery liquid remaining after milk has been curdled and strained during the process of making cheese. (You might have seen it sitting at the top of a container of yogurt. You can pour it off and use it, by the way.) It contains a pool of nutrients and growth factors that stimulate the growth of desirable microorganisms, mainly *Lactobacilli*, in the intestines. Also present in whey are B-complex vitamins B3, B5, B6, B12, and folic acid; minerals calcium, magnesium, and zinc; plus potassium and sodium electrolytes.

Whey is used for making yogurt, kefir, and a variety of fermented fruit and vegetable dishes. You'll find a recipe for making basic whey on page 92, which will be needed for many of the recipes in this book. It's simple and easy to make, and it can be kept frozen for up to three months without harming the beneficial microorganisms. (Any longer, and you risk killing them.) Whey can also be added to other dishes such as soups, smoothies, and salad dressings or topped over steamed vegetables for extra flavor and as a naturally added source of probiotics.

Make the Best Brine

Salt and water (brine) are used in many lacto-fermented food preparations, particularly fruits and vegetables. Salting provides a suitable environment for lactic acid bacteria to thrive, which impart the acid flavor to the food, plus salt draws juices out of foods, which are loaded with trace minerals and other nutrients. Lactic acid bacteria tolerate high salt concentrations—generally at a ratio of 1 teaspoon of salt per 1 cup (235 ml) of water. A recipe for making basic brine can be found on page 92.

Pure unrefined sea salt is the best type to use in all of your fermentations. Chemicals of any variety that are often added to regular table salt, such as sodium iodide, can cause problems with the end result. For example, salt with lime impurities will make the brine cloudy, salt with iron impurities can reduce the acidity of the final product, and salt with magnesium will give fermented foods a bitter taste.

As far as water goes, filtered or bottled water works best. Avoid using chlorinated tap water because this will inhibit fermentation. If tap water is all you have on hand, you can make it chlorine free by first boiling it, then letting it cool again to room temperature. Water affects the metabolic activity of cells (including microbial cells) and influences the conditions that encourage their growth. The amount of water available for the survival of microorganisms is referred to as the water activity. The more pure and less contaminated the water used in fermentation, the greater will be the metabolic activity of the microorganisms to support their growth. In general, bacteria require a fairly high water activity to survive. Too low of a water activity tends to encourage yeasts and fungi to dominate, which can spoil the ferment.

The Benefits of a Slow Soak

Soaking grains, beans, nuts, and seeds overnight before fermenting or cooking them will increase their nutrient value because soaking releases important enzymes that allow your body to more easily digest these foods. They naturally contain enzyme inhibitors that block absorption of protein and essential amino acids and that can inhibit fermentation. Soaking them releases their enzymes by initiating a sprouting process that breaks down the outer hull, thereby increasing nutrients and improving digestibility.

Grains, beans, nuts, and seeds all contain phytates (phytic acid), which blocks phosphorus availability and hinders digestion. Phosphorus, a mineral, is essential to the structure and function of much of the human body. It is best known for its part in the creation of bones and teeth and in the transformation of nutrients to energy. Phosphorus also works with the B-complex vitamins, especially thiamin (B1), which plays a role in the proper functioning of both the digestive system and the nervous system. Both iodine and zinc play an important role in the development and function of the reproductive system and need phosphorous in order for the body to properly use them. Soaking grains, nuts, beans, and seeds overnight in warm water in a warm place with a splash of an enzyme-rich acidic medium such as whey, or a small amount of apple cider vinegar, will release these nutrients while reducing anti-nutrients. Their flavor and texture will also improve. Be sure to discard the soaking water and use only fresh water for your fermentations or before cooking these foods.

For those with gluten intolerance, soaking or fermenting gluten-based grain, such as wheat, rye, barley, and some varieties of oats, makes them more digestible and less problematic. The soaking process neutralizes the phytic acid and other enzyme inhibitors present in these foods that block absorption of essential vitamins and minerals. Soaking them for a few hours or overnight, in warm water or a small amount of apple cider vinegar, helps partially break down the difficult to digest protein, making these grains easier to digest and absorb.

Feed Your Probiotics

Be sure to consume foods that encourage probiotics to flourish. Prebiotic plant foods rich in fiber provide fructooligosaccharides (FOS) and inulin, which feed beneficial bacteria, thus stimulating their growth and providing an environment for them to thrive in your gastrointestinal tract. The best prebiotic foods are raw Jerusalem artichokes, garlic, bananas, chicory root, dandelion root, and wheat bran; raw or lightly steamed asparagus; and raw or cooked onion.

UP THE ANTE ON DAILY FERMENTED FOODS

In addition to preparing recipes from this book or buying already fermented products, you can look for opportunities to increase beneficial flora and prebiotics in meals and recipes. With very little effort you can create a big impact on your health. Apart from their enzymes and probiotics, fermented vegetables added to your meals will naturally boost the nutritional content of the foods they are served with. Beneficial lactic acids increase the bioavailability of vitamins and minerals in other foods by helping break down the food and increase absorption of its nutrients. Lacto-fermented foods can double the digestibility of starches and make fibrous parts more edible.

Use the guide on page 74 to see how you can make simple ingredient substitutions that will give your recipes and meals a flavorsome, healthful boost.

If you're wondering how to introduce or incorporate fermented foods into your daily diet, then you may want to start off with fermented vegetables and add already-prepared ferments to your other dishes. Here are some suggestions for ways to introduce sauerkraut, kimchi, and other assorted fermented vegetables into your daily fare:

- Add sauerkraut to grilled sausages, bratwurst, fish, turkey, and chicken; on mashed potatoes; in mixed salads, potato salad, and coleslaw; in sandwiches, wraps, tacos, enchiladas, rice, beans, tortilla soups, and vegetables of all varieties.

- Add kimchi to rice, beans, wraps, stir-fries, eggs, and braised greens (spinach, kale, collards, Swiss chard), sausages, turkey, and chicken.

- Add tempeh to stir-fry vegetables and braised greens (spinach, kale, collards, Swiss chard), and use as a source of protein in place of meat.

Substitution Guide	
Instead of	**Use**
White flour	Sourdough bread, noodles, sprouted whole-grain versions
Bread crumbs	Sprouted rolled oats or crushed bran
White rice	Brown rice, wild rice, quinoa, bulgur
Commercial cereals	Fermented grains (rolled oats, rice), presoaked granola
Milk or cream	Yogurt, coconut milk
Processed cheese	Mature aged cheeses, seed cheese, goat cheese
Salad dressing	Yogurt, miso, sauerkraut water
Oil-based marinades	Miso, balsamic vinegar, lemon juice, celery juice
Commercial dips	Hummus, guacamole, salsa, with whey culture added
Mayonnaise	Yogurt with sauerkraut water added, herbs
Table salt	Miso, herbs, lemon or lime juice
Margarine	Extra-virgin olive oil, coconut oil, butter, ghee
Garlic	Fermented garlic
Carrot sticks	Fermented carrot sticks
Coleslaw	Fermented carrot and cabbage, with or without added whey
Meats	Tempeh, natto
Fish	Natto sushi
Sugar	Halve the amount, nutmeg, cinnamon, honey

If you decide to incorporate fermented dairy products, consider adding yogurt instead of cream to sauces, marinades, and dips. You can add fruits, such as berries, and a small amount of honey to yogurt, which makes a delicious topping over pies and other desserts, or blend it up for a morning smoothie.

Try these foods and beverages to start:

- yogurt (raw, unpasteurized)
- aged cheese
- sour cream
- crème fraîche
- buttermilk
- kefir
- sauerkraut
- kimchi
- traditionally fermented pickled vegetables: olives, pickles, capers, peppers
- traditionally fermented soy products: miso, tempch, tofuyo (fermented tofu), soy sauce, natto
- traditionally marinated vegetables: artichokes, olives, peppers, mushrooms
- cured meats: sausages, salami, corned beef, pepperoni (nitrate/nitrite free)
- umeboshi plums
- fish sauce
- sourdough bread
- kombucha
- wines (nonalcoholic)
- ciders
- sake

The best fermented foods are raw and unpasteurized, have not been heated, and have been naturally fermented without alcohol or vinegar. Heating foods above approximately 125°F (52°C) destroys live enzymes and prevents the population of beneficial microorganisms. If you purchase pasteurized fermented food products, make sure that they were not pasteurized a second time after fermenting (look for "contains live cultures" on the label).

HOW SOON WILL YOU SEE IMPROVEMENTS?

Many people around the world eat fermented foods at each meal. The Japanese eat miso, and the Koreans eat kimchi with breakfast, lunch, and dinner. Eating probiotic foods regularly is what ensures a healthy abundance of the beneficial microflora. Since having introduced fermented foods into my own diet, and that of my family's, I am noticing more energy, clearer skin and eyes, shinier hair, stronger nails, and reduced weight because the improved absorption of nutrients lessens hunger. But how long it takes for anyone to notice changes is individual.

If consuming fermented foods is new to you, then moderation is the way to go. Start by introducing them gradually into your diet to allow your body time to adjust. Because many people are deficient in beneficial bacteria and digestive enzymes, fermented foods may cause changes in your digestive system shortly after eating them. Mild bloating and gas, for example, are normal and healthy reactions as your body gets accustomed to the changes in your diet. This will go away after your body is restored to a more balanced and efficient mode of digestion and as your friendly microflora builds. If you experience gas or bloating or other similar symptoms, start with one spoonful of the fermented food per day while rebuilding digestive health.

If you are sensitive to molds and yeast or you have a chronic candida infection, you may need to use caution or avoid consuming foods with high mold or yeast content, including some cheeses, vinegar, fruit wines, mushrooms, and fermented soy such as miso, natto, or tempeh.

Lactic acid–producing fermentations should be less problematic. Once your body has built up a healthy population of microflora, any adverse reactions will be significantly diminished and less likely to pose problems.

When excess yeast, viral, and bacterial organisms in the body die off, they release toxins that the body has to then process and eliminate. This can result in an immune reaction if it happens too rapidly for the body to handle. The candida yeast cells are known to release several toxins; among them are ethanol and acetaldehyde, which can cause detrimental effects to health, including impaired brain function, endocrine disruption, and affected immune and respiratory function. Symptoms such as brain fog, fatigue, headache, dizziness, joint aches or muscle pains, itchy skin, hives, rashes, and skin breakouts can all be the result of this die-off. Quite often the liver pathways have been overwhelmed during the elimination process. In a normal effort to detoxify the toxins and poisons, the body reacts by creating inflammatory symptoms. Such symptoms normally pass within a week or so and do not warrant that you stop eating fermented foods altogether. Taking additional probiotics often helps, as does increasing water intake to flush toxins faster through liver detox pathways, and increasing your intake of vitamin C.

If you are on a low-sodium diet, be aware that some commercially fermented foods, such as capers and olives, can be high in salt. If salt is an issue, you may want to stick to fermenting your own foods, where you have more control over the process and can use high-quality mineral salts that do not contain sodium iodide because these are not as problematic.

MAKING FERMENTED FOODS
A FAMILY AFFAIR

A considerable portion of your nutritional needs can be met through fermented foods and beverages. This makes them an ideal choice to include every day in at least one meal, or more whenever possible. Many people enjoy the sour, pungent taste of fermented foods from the first mouthful, whereas for others they are an acquired taste. Introducing these foods to your family may be a challenge, but the rewards and health benefits are well worth the effort.

Perhaps one of the more difficult changes will be for your taste buds, which have become accustomed to a sweeter-tasting diet than one that includes sour, salty, and pungent flavors. One of the biggest factors affecting our modern diets is the amount of sugar we consume because it's added to so many products. Reducing the amount of candy, cakes, and desserts we eat is only part of the solution. Large amounts of added sugar can be hidden in foods such as bread, dairy products, frozen dinners, fast food, canned soups and vegetables, breakfast cereals, salad dressing, and ketchup. These foods all lack vitamins, minerals, and essential fatty acids and contain empty calories, all of which in the end drive us to crave and consume even more sugar.

Although it's good to have a little sweetness in your life, there is a downside to eating too much sugar that far outweighs any short-term benefits. If you crave sugar, there's a big chance you have an imbalance in your gut flora. Sugar feeds pathogenic bacteria and provides them with an opportunity to thrive and dominate. The good news is that the lactic acid and unique flavors in fermented foods actually have a balancing effect that instantly neutralizes sugar cravings. In fact, if you eat sugary foods and follow them up with fermented ones, the beneficial flora in the fermented foods will immediately begin eating up the sugar, minimizing the amount of sugar that your body actually digests.

Shortly after you eat sugary foods, the excess sugar in your body causes blood sugar levels to rise rapidly. This creates a sudden increase in insulin and often leads to reactive hypoglycemia whereby blood sugar levels dip too low. Once this happens your body will naturally crave more sugar in an effort to raise blood sugar and glucose levels back to a stable level. With this unhealthy cycle comes a host of symptoms ranging from excess fat storage (which may eventually lead to diabetes), low energy, brain fog, and irritability.

Introducing children to fermented foods can be challenging because they are less inclined to eat vegetables or "strange" foods, and they often have become accustomed to eating sweets and sugary cereals at breakfast. Many packaged breakfast cereals consist mostly of highly refined rice, corn, or wheat, all of which rapidly convert into glucose in the body. In fact, some brands of breakfast cereals contain more sugar in one bowl than in a similar portion of cake or ice cream. In addition, the process of refining the starches and carbohydrates in packaged foods robs them of important minerals, such as chromium, calcium, phosphorus, iron, and magnesium, along with vitamins A, C, and B complex. These nutrients are the ones most needed for healthy growth, repair, and maintenance within a child's growing body.

To successfully transition your children toward eating fermented foods every day, you should do it in a few gradual steps. For example, start them off at breakfast with homemade, good-quality muesli that contains presoaked grains, fresh fruits, and lacto-fermented yogurt. Instead of white flour pancakes, make sourdough ones and top them with yogurt, fruit, and a teaspoon of honey. The idea is to start getting their taste buds accustomed to the tarter, more sour taste of fermented foods with less sweetness. Here are some other fermented foods they might like:

- plain yogurt mixed with naturally sweetened fresh fruit, such as berries or orange slices

- fermented cheeses with apple slices; tempeh slices; sourdough with fermented fruit jam and cheese; or fermented hummus or avocado dips for snacks

- smoothies made with fresh fermented berries and yogurt

- hot dogs with fermented meats and sauerkraut, served with homemade lacto-fermented relishes or ketchup

Even if you have to strike a deal or bribe them into having at least one bite, or sneak fermented foods into their regular dishes, eventually your children will learn to love them. Involve your children in the fermenting process and watch their delight as they learn about microorganisms in foods they eat and how they work to support health. Gradually, they will begin to crave these foods in their diet as their system adjusts and they associate how much better they feel after eating them. As an added bonus, there will be less time spent on doctors' visits and more time to focus on the creative things they enjoy doing.

You can take heart in knowing that fermentation is one of the oldest food-processing technologies in the world. For generations, the process has been passed down from parent to child. Fermenting your own foods at home is fun and easy to do. Just about any food can be fermented or cultured to increase its nutritional value and to preserve it for months after harvest. And somehow, foods you prepare yourself are often tastier, perhaps because they are made with more love and tender care. You can shop for and include farm-fresh ingredients that have been grown locally and spend only a fraction of the cost that you would with store-bought foods.

Pick a food that you and your family already eat, perhaps yogurt, as your first food or fermentation project. It's simple and easy to do—all you need is milk and some starter culture, and within a few hours you will have yogurt! Add some fresh fruit and eat it as a snack or dessert. From there you can ferment fruits and vegetables by soaking them in brine, and in less than a week, you will have a tasty, inexpensive, and probiotic-rich food. Add starter cultures to mayonnaise, ketchup, and other condiments to make them more nourishing. Let them sit out at room temperature, covered, for a few hours, then refrigerate. The food will be much tastier and you'll know that it has been blessed with a healthy dose of love.

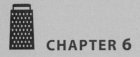

CHAPTER 6

Meal Plans for Common Disorders

"While we may not be able to control all that happens to us,
we can control what happens inside us."

— BENJAMIN FRANKLIN

From a holistic point of view, healing any part of the body must begin with a view of the body as a single integrated system in which all parts are designed to function in a unified manner. Keep in mind that proper digestion plays a critical role in the natural healing process of the entire body because the constant renewal of cells is dependent on proper digestive functioning to extract nutrients that support overall physical and mental health.

No part of your body exists in isolation from any other part. View your body as a whole organism with an organic connection that exists among all tissues, organs, and structures. When you bring healing to any one organ system of your body, you naturally strengthen and heal other systems.

In this chapter I've provided simple meal plan suggestions to launch your journey. Restoration, repair, and rebalancing of your metabolism, strengthening of your immune and digestive systems, easy weight loss, and elimination of food cravings (especially sugary carbohydrates) can soon follow as a natural result.

With that said, all of the fermented food suggestions listed in each of the meal plans below will benefit your entire health. Although they're mapped out by day and by meal, the menu suggestions are interchangeable for any meal. The idea is to increase your daily, regular consumption of fermented foods, starting with breakfast, and to focus on eating a variety of foods from all of the main food groups to include fresh and fermented fruits, vegetables, grains, legumes, and meats and fish (if you're not vegetarian). Soon you will experience increased energy levels, fewer aches and pains, reduced weight (or increased weight, if that's what your body needs), and stronger immunity. You may even notice that symptoms you thought you would simply have to live with have completely vanished.

CONQUERING DIGESTIVE DISORDERS

High-fiber foods such as vegetables, fruits, beans, and cereal grains all help keep waste materials moving through your small and large intestines at a healthy pace. High-fiber foods are also prebiotic, which promotes growth of probiotics. And of course, all fermented foods will naturally enhance probiotic population and nutrient absorption, and help to conquer digestive disorders. Remember to drink plenty of water in between meals to flush your colon and cleanse your kidneys. Choose any dishes from the following suggestions.

Meal Plan for Conquering Digestive Disorders

Monday
Breakfast Soaked-grain muesli or granola with yogurt and Fermented Mango, Cinnamon, and Peach Chutney (page 114)

Lunch Russian Cucumber-Kefir Soup (page 152)

Snack Sprouted tortilla chips with Stomach-Soothing Tzatziki Herb Sauce (page 160)

Dinner Stir-fry using soaked grains or legumes with vegetables, and meat or tempeh

Tuesday
Breakfast Refreshing Orange Coconut Kefir Smoothie (page 158), made with papaya and berries

Lunch Raw salad made with spinach or dark, leafy lettuce, avocado, tomato, sprouts, onions, celery, carrots, and bell peppers, topped with Yogurt Kefir Ranch Dip (page 161) as a dressing

Snack Energy-Boosting Granola Bars (page 146)

Dinner Fish of your choice, served with Digestive Orange, Ginger, and Raisin Relish (page 174) and Protein-Powered Pinto Beans (page 146)

Sprouting Chips

The demand for sprouted grain products is on the rise, and it's becoming easier to find more variety and options available at supermarkets. To make sprouted tortilla chips, you can simply buy sprouted tortillas and make them into chips by cutting them, lightly coating or spritzing them with olive oil, then baking them in a 350°F (180°C, or gas mark 4) oven, turning once, about 10 minutes, or until crisp. There are a couple of companies, such as Ezekiel and Garden of Eatin's, making them from a sprouted grain combination of brown rice, lentils, and quinoa. These are great if you're avoiding gluten.

Wednesday

Breakfast Sprouted Enzymatic Brown Rice (page 130) served with Plum Yum Prune Sauce (page 116)

Lunch Simple Sauerkraut (page 93) added to whatever you're having for lunch, with a side of Garlic Dill Pickles Delight (page 112)

Snack Easy Kefir Cheese (page 148) served with sprouted crackers or raw vegetables

Dinner Wholesome Tempeh Burgers (page 144) topped with Must-Have Honey-Dill Mustard (page 177) and served with Anti-Inflammatory Apple and Juniper Berry Kraut (page 94)

Thursday

Breakfast For-the-Love-of-Sourdough Bread (page 135), or Symbiotic Sourdough Pancakes (page 136), served with Digestive Pineapple Chutney (page 122)

Lunch Pickled or fermented meats served with fermented condiments, such as Digestive Pickled Radishes with Ginger and Apple (page 110)

Snack Garlic Dill Pickles Delight (page 112)

Dinner Your choice of fish, chicken, or beef served with Detoxifying Pickled Turnips and Beets (page 97)

Friday

Breakfast Two scrambled or poached eggs or omelet with Prebiotic Vegetable Medley Kraut (page 98)

Lunch Raw salad greens served with Probiotic-Rich Radish Kimchi (page 100) and fermented salad dressing

Snack Digestive Lemon-Ginger Kombucha (page 186)

Dinner Easily Digestible Pizza Dough (page 138) served with your choice of toppings

Saturday

Breakfast Enzyme-Potent Papaya-Cinnamon Kombucha Smoothie (page 116)

Lunch Stress-Less Gazpacho (page 111), or a mixed leafy green salad with salmon, turkey, or chicken, and fermented dressing (page 83)

Snack Fermented yogurt combined with fruit

Dinner Sourdough wraps, tacos, pizza, or sandwiches, served with assorted fermented vegetables

Sunday

Breakfast Yogurt mixed with Apple, Ginger, and Mint Chutney with a Kick (page 122) topped over sprouted granola

Lunch Immune-Building Miso Soup with Tofu (page 135), or a mixed leafy green salad with salmon, turkey, or chicken, and fermented dressing (page 83)

Snack Simple Sauerkraut (page 93)

Dinner Your choice of fish, beef, chicken, or turkey served with Cleansing Beets with Ginger and Grapefruit (page 105)

BOOSTING YOUR IMMUNE SYSTEM

Salmon, salads, smoothies, antioxidants, spices, and supplements such as zinc and omega-3s are the top nutritional choices for boosting your immune system. Colorful foods, such as tomatoes, blueberries, beetroot, carrots, and strawberries, are all high in antioxidants that strengthen the immune system. Include raw garlic in your daily diet because this flavorful member of the onion family stimulates the multiplication of infection-fighting white cells, boosts natural killer cell activity, and increases the efficiency of antibody production. Zinc, found in beef, turkey, beans, legumes, and cereals, increases the production of white blood cells that fight infection. Fermentation increases all of these important immune-boosting nutrients. Choose any dish from the following suggestions.

Meal Plan for Boosting Your Immune System

Monday
Breakfast Kefir smoothie made with fruits such as papaya, pineapple, and berries

Lunch Mixed leafy green salad served with salmon, turkey, or chicken, and Simple Sauerkraut (page 93), or Immune-Building Miso Soup with Tofu (page 135)

Snack Sprouted tortilla chips served with Strengthening Spinach Hummus (page 139)

Dinner Your choice of fish, chicken, beef, or tempeh garnished with Unforgettable Pickled Garlic with Rosemary and Lemon (page 96)

Tuesday
Breakfast Soaked-grain muesli or granola with yogurt and Tropical Coconut, Mango, and Mint Chutney (page 126)

Lunch Mixed leafy green salad combined with quinoa, salmon, turkey, or chicken, and onions, ginger, garlic, and fermented dressing (page 83)

Snack Refreshing Kombucha Tea (page 181), or Lacto-Fermented Lemons or Limes (page 118)

Dinner Weight-Reducing Tempeh Coconut Curry (page 132)

Wednesday
Breakfast Blueberry kefir smoothie

Lunch Mixed leafy green salad combined with spinach, onions, tomatoes, sauerkraut, and Infection-Fighting Fermented Chili Sauce (page 177)

Snack Raw veggies served with Yogurt Kefir Ranch Dip (page 161)

Dinner Your choice of tempeh, quinoa, fish, chicken, or beef, served with fermented vegetable of your choice

Thursday
Breakfast Two-egg omelet with tomatoes and served with Simple Sauerkraut (page 93)

Lunch Mixed leafy green salad combined with spinach, avocado, sauerkraut, and Unforgettable Pickled Garlic with Rosemary and Lemon (page 96)

Snack Revitalizing Rejuvelac (page 182) or Refreshing Kombucha Tea (page 181)

Dinner Your choice of tempeh, quinoa, fish, or chicken, served with Antioxidant-Rich Asparagus Spears (page 106)

Friday

Breakfast Soaked-grain muesli or granola, with yogurt and fermented fruit chutney (Chapter 8)

Lunch Mixed leafy green salad combined with radishes, beets, carrots, and Immune-Boosting Onion and Bell Pepper Relish or fermented salad dressing (below)

Snack Kefir smoothie with berries of your choice

Dinner Your choice of fish, beef, or chicken, served with steamed asparagus and broccoli and Simple Sauerkraut (page 93)

Simple Salad Dressing

You can greatly improve your digestion by eating fermented salad dressing, which you can literally whip up in seconds. In a screw-top jar, simply add a couple tablespoons of apple cider vinegar, the same amount of lemon juice, a doubled amount of extra-virgin olive oil (or combine one-half flaxseed oil with one-half olive oil), and 1 teaspoon mustard powder; pour some of the juice from your sauerkraut into the concoction. Place the lid on tightly and shake vigorously. You've made a dressing that not only tastes delicious but is also a homemade digestive aid. Eat it daily, and remember to pour it over your steamed vegetables, too.

Saturday

Breakfast Two scrambled, boiled, or poached eggs served with grapefruit and berries and Energizing Green Tea Kombucha (page 185)

Lunch Mixed leafy green salad combined with avocado, tomatoes, and tuna, salmon, or chicken, and Garlic Dill Pickles Delight (page 112)

Snack Hydrating Coconut Water (page 188) or Blood-Purifying Beet Kvass (page 187)

Dinner Brain-Protective Honey-Ginger Salmon (page 164) served with steamed broccoli and asparagus

Sunday

Breakfast Symbiotic Sourdough Pancakes (page 136) served with Plum Yum Prune Sauce (page 116)

Lunch Mixed leafy green salad combined with avocado and Ginger-Carrot Kraut (page 102)

Snack Cooling Carrot and Celery Kefir (page 154)

Dinner Strengthening Herbed Corned Beef (page 166) or Dynamic Baked Beans (page 140) served with steamed asparagus and cauliflower

REPAIRING YOUR METABOLISM

Low-calorie or starvation diets undertaken for prolonged periods put stress on your metabolism, can cause it to become inefficient, and can damage cells. Eating the right foods at regular intervals throughout the day, avoiding the wrong foods (such as sugar, white flour, processed carbohydrates, and trans fats), avoiding toxins, and keeping your hormones balanced are the keys to repairing a damaged metabolism. Sprouted and fermented whole grains, legumes, nuts, and seeds; colorful fruits and vegetables; and organic fermented dairy products, meats, fish, and eggs eaten throughout the day can boost a weakened metabolism. Eat a hearty breakfast—never skip this important meal!—and eat fermented snacks between meals. Doing so will prevent hunger pangs and provide consistent energy to maintain metabolism efficiency. Sprinkle some fermented foods into your meals, even if it is only a bite or two, and you'll repair and keep your immune system strong and healthy. Keep your body well hydrated throughout the day with water and probiotic tonics and beverages. Choose any dish from the following suggestions.

Meal Plan for Repairing Your Metabolism

Monday

Breakfast Fermented grains or beans or two eggs prepared any style with avocado and tomato

Snack Blood-Purifying Beet Kvass (page 187), Refreshing Kombucha Tea (page 181), or Revitalizing Rejuvelac (page 182)

Lunch Mixed leafy green salad served with your choice of fish, chicken, or tempeh, with grated carrots, sauerkraut, and black olives, and Must-Have Honey-Dill Mustard (page 177)

Snack Cleansing Probiotic Limonade (page 190), Blood-Purifying Beet Kvass (page 187), or Refreshing Kombucha Tea (page 181)

Dinner Love-Your-Heart Lentil Dal (page 143), served with your choice of fish, chicken, or beef, and add some steamed broccoli, cauliflower, and asparagus (or other fresh seasonal leafy green vegetable)

Tuesday

Breakfast Choice of soaked-grain muesli or granola with yogurt and fermented fruit chutney or two eggs any style, with grapefruit and berries

Snack Revitalizing Rejuvelac (page 182), Energizing Green Tea Kombucha (page 185), or Hydrating Coconut Water (page 188)

Lunch Enzyme-Powered Natto Sushi Rolls (page 128) served with Plum Yum Prune Sauce (page 116), or a large leafy green salad with carrots, tomato, avocado, and sauerkraut

Snack Energy-Boosting Granola Bars (page 146), or Wild Mixed Berries Frozen Yogurt (page 162)

Dinner Protein-Powered Pinto Beans (page 146), served with your choice of fish, chicken, turkey, or beef and Antioxidant-Rich Asparagus Spears (page 106)

Wednesday

Breakfast Your choice of Dynamic Baked Beans (page 140), two eggs any style served with fermented vegetables of your choice, or Refreshing Orange Coconut Kefir Smoothie (page 158) with added berries

Snack Refreshing Kombucha Tea (page 181), Cleansing Probiotic Limonade (page 190), or Blood-Purifying Beet Kvass (page 187)

Lunch Mixed leafy green salad combined with spinach, carrot, avocado, and sauerkraut, and your choice of fish, chicken, or turkey, or Love-Your-Heart Lentil Dal (page 143)

Snack Energy-Boosting Granola Bars (page 146)

Dinner Weight-Reducing Tempeh Coconut Curry (page 132)

Soak All Grains, Nuts, and Seeds

Grains, nuts, and seeds are not always easy to digest because their skin contains an enzyme inhibitor called phytic acid that prevents them from releasing their beneficial nutrients. Phytic acid prevents premature germination and stores nutrients for plant growth, which is great for the plant, but it also inhibits your digestion and absorption. The easy way to get around this is to soak all nuts and seeds in purified water first before fermenting or eating them, just as you would do with beans and grains (remember to toss out the soaking water before fermenting or cooking them). By soaking your nuts and seeds overnight, you release the enzyme inhibitors and essentially activate the growth process, which allows your body to absorb their nutrients. Rinse them well after soaking and toss out the soaking water. See page 72, in chapter 5, for more information.

Thursday

Breakfast Your choice of two eggs any style, served with Cleansing Beets with Ginger and Grapefruit (page 105)

Snack Energy-Boosting Granola Bars (page 146)

Lunch Mixed leafy green salad with spinach, black olives, carrot, and sauerkraut, and served with your choice of fish, chicken, turkey, or tempeh

Snack Refreshing Kombucha Tea (page 181), or Cleansing Probiotic Limonade (page 191), or Blood-Purifying Beet Kvass (page 187)

Dinner Lacto-Fermented Lentils (page 131) served with Fermented Mediterranean Mackerel (page 168)

Friday

Breakfast Yogurt with Plum Yum Prune Sauce (page 116), or Refreshing Orange Coconut Kefir Smoothie (page 158)

Snack Russian Cucumber-Kefir Soup (page 152), or Fermented Virgin Mary with a Twist (page 190)

Lunch Mixed leafy green salad combined with spinach, black olives, carrot, and sauerkraut, and served with your choice of fish, chicken, turkey, or tempeh; or Strengthening Spinach Hummus (page 139) served with sprouted tortilla chips

Snack Cooling Carrot and Celery Kefir (page 154), or Wild Mixed Berries Frozen Yogurt (page 162)

Dinner Protein-Powered Pinto Beans (page 146) served with your choice of fish, chicken, turkey, beef, or tempeh, lightly stir-fried or baked

Saturday

Breakfast Your choice of two eggs any style served with Enzyme-Rich Tomatillo and Mint Salsa (page 108), or soaked-grain muesli or granola with yogurt and fermented fruit chutney (Chapter 8) or relish (Chapter 11)

Snack Refreshing Kombucha Tea (page 181), Cleansing Probiotic Limonade (page 190), Blood-Purifying Beet Kvass (page 187), or Revitalizing Rejuvelac (page 182)

Lunch Stress-Less Gazpacho (page TK), or sprouted tortilla chips served with fermented avocado, hummus, or Stomach-Soothing Tzatziki Herb Sauce (page 160)

Snack Yogurt with fresh fruit, or Energy-Boosting Granola Bars (page 146)

Dinner Wholesome Tempeh Burgers (page 144) served with Prebiotic Vegetable Medley Kraut (page 98) or steamed veggies

Sunday

Breakfast Soaked-grain muesli or granola with yogurt and fermented fruit chutney (Chapter 8) or relish (Chapter 11), or omelet served with Cleansing Beets with Ginger and Grapefruit (page 105)

Snack Refreshing Kombucha Tea (page 181), Cleansing Probiotic Limonade (page 190), Blood-Purifying Beet Kvass (page 182), or Revitalizing Rejuvelac (page 182)

Lunch Mixed leafy green salad combined with spinach, black olives, and carrot, and sauerkraut, and your choice of fish, chicken, turkey, or tempeh; or Immune-Building Miso Soup with Tofu (page 135)

Snack Energy-Boosting Granola Bars (page 146)

Dinner Sprouted Enzymatic Brown Rice (page 130) served with tempeh, fish, or chicken

REGULATING WEIGHT AND REDUCING CRAVINGS

Maintaining stable blood sugar levels throughout the day helps eliminate cravings for unhealthful foods and is the key to healthy weight loss. Eating fermented foods makes essential nutrients more easily available for the body to use, allowing you to feel more satisfied and comfortably eat less. This prevents spikes in blood sugar and creates an inner nutritional balance that both halts food cravings and supports weight loss. And, as an added benefit, fermented foods' sour taste—the exact opposite of sweet—can stop sugar cravings in their tracks! Be sure to include a small amount of protein at your three main meals each day as this ensures your metabolism will be well fueled to help you to burn fat more easily. Choose any dish from the following suggestions and feel free to mix them up as you like.

Meal Plan for Regulating Weight and Reducing Cravings

Monday
Breakfast Two-egg omelet with Enzyme-Rich Tomatillo and Mint Salsa (page 108)

Lunch Detoxifying Pickled Turnips and Beets (page 97), served with a mixed green leafy salad containing either fish, chicken, turkey, or beef

Snack Refreshing Kombucha Tea (page 181), Cleansing Probiotic Limonade (page 190), Blood-Purifying Beet Kvass (page 187), or Revitalizing Rejuvelac (page 182)

Dinner Weight-Reducing Tempeh Coconut Curry (page 132)

Tuesday
Breakfast Soaked-grain muesli or granola with yogurt and Probiotic Berry Good-for-You Jam (page 121), or two eggs any style served with fermented vegetables of your choice

Lunch Mixed leafy green salad combined with spinach, carrot, and sauerkraut, and served with your choice of fish, chicken, turkey, or tempeh with Digestive Pickled Radishes with Ginger and Apple (page 110)

Snack Refreshing Kombucha Tea (page 181), Cleansing Probiotic Limonade (page 190), Blood-Purifying Beet Kvass (page 187), or Revitalizing Rejuvelac (page 182)

Dinner Your choice of fish, chicken, beef, or turkey served with Ginger-Carrot Kraut (page 102)

Wednesday

Breakfast Yogurt served with Cleansing Beets with Ginger and Grapefruit (page 105), or two eggs any style served with Simple Sauerkraut (page 93)

Lunch Mixed leafy green salad combined with spinach, carrot, and sauerkraut, and your choice of fish, chicken, turkey, or tempeh, served with Probiotic-Rich Radish Kimchi (page 100)

Snack Fermented Virgin Mary with a Twist (page 190), Refreshing Kombucha Tea (page 181), or Cleansing Probiotic Limonade (page 190)

Dinner Enzyme-Powered Natto Sushi Rolls (page 128), served with leafy green salad and carrots

Thursday

Breakfast Soaked-grain muesli or granola with yogurt and Probiotic Berry Good-for-You Jam (page 121), or two eggs any style served with fermented vegetables of your choice

Lunch A mixed leafy green salad combined with spinach, carrot, and sauerkraut, and served with your choice of fish, chicken, turkey, or tempeh with Must-Have Honey-Dill Mustard (page 177)

Snack Fermented Virgin Mary with a Twist (page 190), Refreshing Kombucha Tea (page 181), or Cleansing Probiotic Limonade (page 190)

Dinner Protein-Powered Pinto Beans (page 146), with either Prebiotic Vegetable Medley Kraut (page 98) or steamed broccoli, cauliflower, and asparagus

Making Yogurt

To make yogurt, simply add 2 to 3 tablespoons (30–45 ml) whey or store-bought plain yogurt to 1 pint (473 ml) of milk. (Make sure the label on store-bought yogurt says the product contains "live active cultures," though, as some brands pasteurize the product after it's been made.) Set out at room temperature overnight, and in the morning, you'll have yogurt!

Homemade yogurt is not only cheaper than store-bought yogurt, but it is also simple to make, and it tastes so much better. Making it requires no special equipment (other than a thermometer to ensure the temperature stays consistent at around 100°F [38°C] to encourage bacterial growth). Homemade yogurt contains more beneficial probiotics and doesn't have the added sugar or chemicals, or produce the packaging waste of store-bought yogurt. Be sure to use whole milk for a creamier, thicker texture, or if it's available, raw milk makes the yogurt even creamier and more healthful.

Friday

Breakfast Soaked-grain muesli or granola with yogurt and Probiotic Berry Good-for-You Jam (page 121), or two eggs any style served with fermented vegetables of your choice

Lunch Russian Cucumber-Kefir Soup (page 152), or a mixed leafy green salad combined with spinach, carrot, and sauerkraut, and served with your choice of fish, chicken, turkey, or tempeh with Heart-Healthy Mayonnaise (page 176)

Snack Fermented Virgin Mary with a Twist (page 190), Refreshing Kombucha Tea (page 181), or Cleansing Probiotic Limonade (page 190)

Dinner Artery-Protective Pickled Herring (page 170), served with steamed broccoli, cabbage, and asparagus

Saturday

Breakfast Soaked-grain muesli or granola with yogurt and Probiotic Berry Good-for-You Jam (page 121), or two eggs any style served with fermented vegetables of your choice

Lunch Stress-Less Gazpacho (page 111), or a mixed leafy green salad combined with spinach, carrot, and sauerkraut, and your choice of fish, chicken, turkey, or tempeh served with Cleansing Beet and Apple Relish (page 174)

Snack Fermented Virgin Mary with a Twist (page 190), Refreshing Kombucha Tea (page 181), or Cleansing Probiotic Limonade (page 190)

Dinner Artery-Protective Pickled Herring (page 170), served with steamed broccoli, cabbage, and asparagus

Sunday

Breakfast Soaked-grain muesli or granola with yogurt and Probiotic Berry Good-for-You Jam (page 121), or two eggs any style served with fermented vegetables of your choice

Lunch Stomach-Soothing Tzatziki Herb Sauce (page 160) served with sprouted tortilla chips

Snack Refreshing Kombucha Tea (page 181), Cleansing Probiotic Limonade (page 190), Blood-Purifying Beet Kvass (page 187), or Revitalizing Rejuvelac (page 182)

Dinner Wholesome Tempeh Burgers (page 144) with Simple Sauerkraut (page 93)

OPTIMUM HEALTH IS WITHIN REACH

Keep colonizing your gastrointestinal tract with regular daily consumption of fermented foods used as probiotic therapy. Doing so will ensure restoration of your internal ecosystem. Other benefits include clearer, smoother skin, more pleasant breath, sweeter-smelling bowel movements, and feelings of calmness and balance as your body becomes more nourished.

Explore the recipes in the next section and experiment with making your own delicious fermented foods at home. I've included a sampling of some of my favorite recipes, but there's no end to the combinations that can be created from fermenting foods.

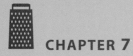

CHAPTER 7

Vegetables

Growing up with a European dad meant that fermented food was a part of our daily diet. For the most part, it included such foods as raw fermented sauerkraut, fermented beets, pickled dill cucumbers, and pickled herring, all of which were added to just about every meal we ate (except breakfast). It certainly was a far cry from what my friends were eating at the time, and I can remember begging my mother not to serve it when they came for dinner for fear of being ridiculed and called names the next day in the school yard. Little did I know that my desire not only to eat but also to create my own fermented foods would come full circle.

Born from a desire to nurture good health, prevent disease, and in some cases to cure it, I've changed my eating habits and those of my family. And with that desire, so, too, has my way of preparing and cooking food changed. Fermented foods are simply a part of my everyday diet and life now, and I am always looking for ways to incorporate them into a meal to boost both prebiotic and probiotic content.

In part 3, I share a few family favorites—dishes that are simple and easy to prepare, while providing a colorful array of flavors, textures, and aromas. Preparing fermented foods at home is really an inexact art at best, so don't worry if you're just starting out. I promise that you will soon discover, as I did, that fermenting is super easy and simple, and with each dish you prepare, the benefits, both in taste and health, are worth it. Use these recipes as guidelines and feel free to experiment by creating your own wonderful dishes. There's no shortage of which foods can be fermented and which other foods they can be eaten with.

You'll notice that some of the recipes call for a tight or airlocked lid, while others call for one that is not tight fitting. You can ferment the foods more or less the same way: using tight or not tight. Traditionally, ferments were produced both in airlocked systems and in open systems. Using an airlock reduces the likelihood that your ferment will be contaminated by molds. I almost always use an airlock in fermenting because it is great to use; however, it is not necessary for proper fermentation. A loose seal will help when you need to use yeasts (such as in kombucha and sourdough) and when you don't want your ferment to become bubbly. The real key is that whatever you are fermenting, the solids must rest below the level of the brine.

The fermented vegetables in this chapter provide some of the basic selections to include with your salads, sandwiches, meats, and grain dishes. You can store them in the refrigerator, where they will keep for months and allow you to eat seasonal foods year-round. All vegetables contain essential vitamins, minerals, and fiber—all of which are enhanced through fermentation—with the added benefit of a healthy dose of probiotics. Feel free to experiment with herbs and spices, and you can also add more or less salt depending on your taste.

Easy Whey

Whey is used as a starter culture for creating many of the recipes in this book. Making whey is simple. You'll need some basic equipment, such as a colander, some cheesecloth, and a bowl, along with some fermented dairy to get you started. I like to prepare a few jars to keep on hand at all times. You can use store-bought yogurt if you prefer, but make sure it's made from whole milk rather than low-fat or skim milk, because it's much thicker.

1   quart (946 ml) plain probiotic-rich yogurt, kefir, or other low-temperature fermented dairy

Line a colander with cheesecloth and place it in a large glass bowl. Pour the yogurt into the cheesecloth. Let it drip for a few hours, then tie up the ends of the cheesecloth. Continue letting the whey drip out into the bowl, set out on the counter overnight, then pour the whey into a clean glass jar with a tight-fitting lid. (The white creamy remains in the colander is similar to cream cheese and can be used to spread over toast.) Store in the refrigerator for several weeks, but discard any mold or floating bits in it that might form during storage. Whey may also be frozen for several months, but not indefinitely because organisms perish over time when frozen.

Yield: 2 cups (475 ml)

> *Note   Add whey to your homemade sauces, salad dressings, smoothies, soups, grains, beans, and vegetable and fruit recipes to make them tastier, healthier, and probiotic rich.*

Basic Brine

Many of the foods in the recipes that follow need to be submerged in brine. Brine is super simple to make because it contains only two ingredients: salt and water. The salt tenderizes meats and vegetables and holds back the pathogenic bacteria, allowing the friendly organisms to take over and work their magic.

6   tablespoons (108 g) fine sea salt, or 9 (162 g) tablespoons coarse sea salt

2   quarts (2 L) water, filtered or purified

In a large bowl, combine the salt and water. If the brine is needed immediately, dissolve the salt in a few cups of warm water over heat, then add cold water to make the full 2 quarts. Otherwise, you can make the brine in advance and store it in a glass jar with an airtight lid in the refrigerator. Keeps indefinitely.

Yield: 2 quarts (2 L)

> *Note   When you're ready to use your brine, place the items you want to ferment in a jar, pour the brine over the food, leaving space 1 inch (2.5 cm) from the top, and then seal the jar.*

Simple Sauerkraut

Sauerkraut, which means "sour cabbage," originated in Europe and consists of lacto-fermented cabbage. Cabbage is the most frequently lacto-fermented vegetable, probably because the result tastes so good.

4   **heads red or green cabbage, shredded**

¼   **cup (72 g) fine sea salt, divided**

    Basic Brine (page 92), as needed

Place the cabbage in a large bowl a handful at a time and sprinkle with half the salt. Repeat until all of the cabbage has been salted in the bowl. Add the salted cabbage to a wide-mouth glass fermentation jar or crock, massaging and pressing it down as you go. Liquid will begin to seep from the cabbage. Sprinkle with the rest of the salt. The extracted water should cover the cabbage entirely. If not, add brine to cover. Be sure the level of the liquid stays 1 inch (2.5 cm) below the jar rim to allow for expansion. Press the cabbage down and keep it under the brine by placing a plate or a lid on top, weighted down by a clean rock or resealable plastic bag filled with water.

Leave the jar in a warm, dark spot in your kitchen and allow the sauerkraut to ferment for 7 to 10 days. Check on it from time to time to ensure that the brine still covers the cabbage; add more, if needed. Remove any mold that may form on the surface, and if fruit flies become a problem, cover the jar with a clean towel. A good way to know when it is ready is to taste it during the fermentation process and move it to the refrigerator when you are satisfied with the taste. Make sure to cover it with a lid to preserve nutrients.

Yield: 1 gallon (2.2 kg)

Note   *Sauerkraut is loaded with vitamin C, Lactobacilli, and other nutrients.*

Anti-Inflammatory Apple and Juniper Berry Kraut

The juniper berries lend a unique flavor to this very popular variation on a basic sauerkraut. Known for their reputation as an herbal remedy for a long list of diseases and ailments, juniper berries combine well with cabbage to create a power-packed elixir that explodes with flavor. Use more or less cabbage and apple as your fermenting crock size will allow.

3 or 4 heads red or green cabbage, shredded

2 or 3 apples, peeled, cored, and coarsely chopped

2 tablespoons (13.5 g) caraway seeds

3 tablespoons (23 g) juniper berries, crushed

¼ cup (72 g) fine sea salt, divided

Basic Brine (page 92), as needed

Combine the cabbage, apples, caraway seeds, and juniper berries in a large bowl. Sprinkle with half the salt. Place the mixture, handful by handful, into a fermentation jar or crock; pound vigorously after each addition and sprinkle with the remainder of the salt after each handful. Liquid will begin to seep from the cabbage. The extracted water should cover the cabbage entirely. If not, add brine to cover. Be sure the level of the liquid stays 1 inch (2.5 cm) below the jar rim to allow for expansion. Press the mixture down and keep it under the brine by placing a plate or a lid on top, weighted down by a clean rock or resealable plastic bag filled with water.

Place the fermentation jar in a warm, dark spot in your kitchen and allow the sauerkraut to ferment for 7 to 10 days. Check on it from time to time to ensure that the brine covers the vegetables. Add more if needed. Remove any mold that may form on the surface, and if fruit flies become a problem, cover the crock with a clean towel. A good way to know when it is ready is to taste it during the fermentation process and move it to the refrigerator when you are satisfied with the taste. Keep it covered with a lid.

Yield: 1 gallon (2.2 kg)

Note *Juniper berries have anti-inflammatory and diuretic properties. Because of this they are often of great help to those suffering from arthritis, gout, and rheumatic diseases.*

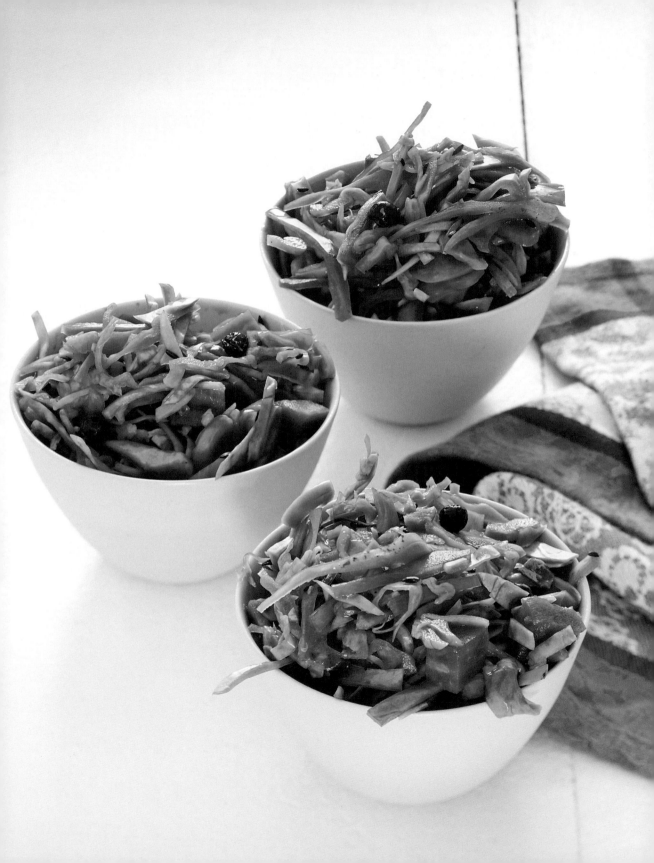

Unforgettable Pickled Garlic with Rosemary and Lemon

Long considered a natural antibiotic in its own right, garlic is well known as an immune booster and anti-inflammatory agent. Its nutritive benefits are increased when you ferment it. Besides adding a balance of soft fragrances to the food, rosemary increases blood flow to the brain and improves memory. You'll love the lemony flavor and high levels of antioxidants in this pickled dish.

4 to 5 heads garlic, cloves separated and peeled

1 teaspoon finely chopped fresh rosemary, or ½ teaspoon dried

¼ teaspoon grated lemon zest

1 teaspoon fine sea salt

¼ cup (60 ml) Easy Whey (page 92)

¼ cup (60 ml) Basic Brine (page 92), or more as needed

In a small bowl, combine the garlic cloves, rosemary, and lemon and sprinkle with salt. Transfer to a fermentation jar and cover with the whey and brine. Place a weight in the jar to ensure that the garlic remains fully submerged. Put a lid loosely on the jar and ferment at room temperature for 7 to 10 days. Screw the lid on tightly and transfer the jar to the refrigerator. The garlic will keep for several months.

Yield: 1 pint (473 ml)

Note Serve as a garnish to salads or add to soups, stir-fries, and dips.

Detoxifying Pickled Turnips and Beets

Teeming with probiotics, fiber, and antioxidants, this combination of turnips and beets is beyond flavorful and will complement any grilled or baked meat dish.

2 or 3 medium turnips, peeled, cut into ¼-inch (6-mm) batons

3 or 4 medium beets, trimmed of greens, peeled, and cut into ¼-inch (6-mm) batons

1 inch (2.5 cm)-long piece fresh ginger, peeled and cut into matchsticks

Zest of 1 orange

2 tablespoons (22 g) mustard seeds, or 1 bay leaf

1 cup (235 ml) Easy Whey (page 92)

Basic Brine (page 92), as needed

In a medium bowl, combine the turnips, beets, ginger, orange zest, and mustard seeds. Place the mixture into a wide-mouth fermenting jar (use two jars if necessary). Pour in the whey to submerge, and add brine, if needed, to cover the mixture. Weight the mixture down, if necessary, and keep it under the brine by placing a plate or a lid on top, weighted down by a clean rock or resealable plastic bag filled with water. Leave the jar in a warm, dark spot in your kitchen and allow the mixture to ferment at room temperature for 3 to 7 days. Check on it periodically to ensure that the brine still covers the vegetables. Screw the lid on tightly and transfer the jar to the refrigerator.

Yield: 1 quart (946 ml)

Turnips and beets are naturally rich in many unique phytonutrients and vitamin C to help boost immunity. Beets are highest in folate, which can prevent neural tube defects in babies when taken by the mother during preconception. Beets also improve liver function largely by thinning the bile, allowing it to flow more freely through the liver and into the small intestine. Together, turnips and beets contain powerful anti-inflammatory and detoxification benefits.

Note Use the ¼-inch (6-mm) blade on a mandoline to cut the peeled vegetables into batons. You can also cut them into ¼-inch (6-mm) rounds if you prefer. Either way, keep the thicknesses the same, as variations in thicknesses can lead to variations in taste and texture.

Prebiotic Vegetable Medley Kraut

Taking sauerkraut a lot further, these vegetable combinations are a great new way to get a variety of superfoods into your daily diet. Because of their fiber content, they will aid digestion and are the perfect complement to every meal. You can spice them up or flavor them with many herbs.

4 apples, cored and diced, with peels left on

4 cups (600 g) cauliflower florets

3 carrots, peeled and diced

6 red onions, thinly sliced

1 cup (67 g) finely chopped kale

3 tablespoons (24 g) grated fresh ginger

¼ cup (72 g) fine sea salt, divided

¼ cup (60 ml) Easy Whey (page 92)

Basic Brine (page 92), as needed

In a large bowl, combine the apples, cauliflower, carrots, onions, kale, and ginger and sprinkle with half the salt. Place the mixture, handful by handful, into a fermentation jar or crock; pound vigorously after each addition and sprinkle each handful with more of the salt. Liquid will begin to seep from the vegetables. Add the whey. The liquid should cover the mixture entirely. If not, add brine to cover. Be sure the level of the liquid stays 1 inch (2.5 cm) below the jar rim to allow for expansion. Press the vegetables down and keep them under the brine by placing a plate or a lid on top, weighted down by a clean rock or resealable plastic bag filled with water.

Leave the jar in a warm, dark spot in your kitchen and allow the vegetables to ferment for 7 to 10 days. Check on it periodically to ensure that the brine still covers the vegetables. Add more brine as needed. Remove any mold that may form on the surface, and if fruit flies become a problem, cover the jar with a clean towel. A good way to know when it is ready is to taste it during the fermentation process and move it to the refrigerator when you are satisfied with the taste. Screw the lid on tightly and transfer the jar to the refrigerator. The veggies will keep for months in the refrigerator.

Yield: About 2 quarts (568 g)

Note *Feel free to experiment using fresh seasonal vegetables for your mixed ferments.*

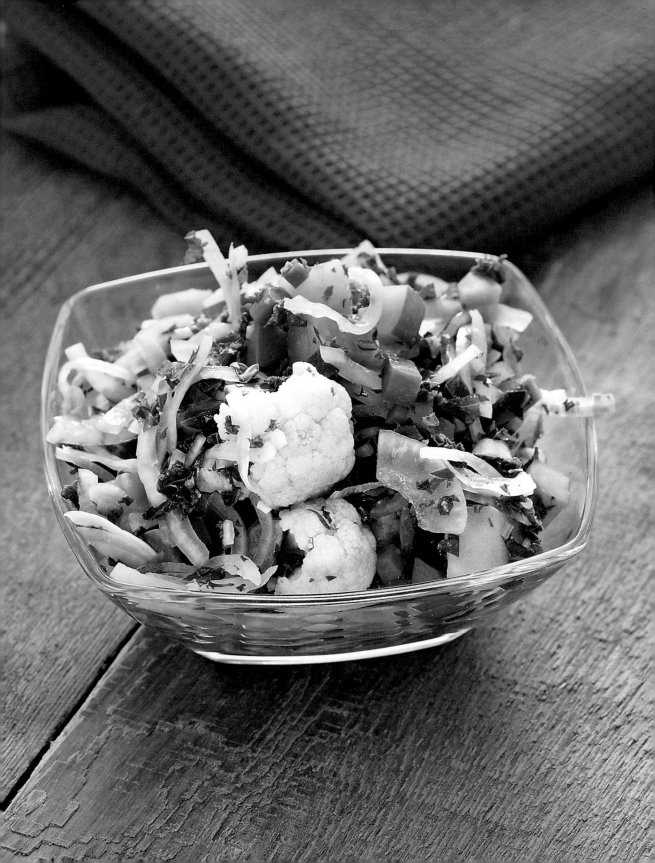

Probiotic-Rich Radish Kimchi

There's no shortage of health benefits from this Korean cousin to sauerkraut. Kimchi is a very spicy and pungent fermented combination of Napa cabbage, radishes, and spicy flavorings. The addition of Asian pear lends a subtle sweetness to its sharp taste. Asian pears are cousins to the pears that are typically seen in grocery stores, but this fruit is similar to an apple in shape. Other names this pear goes by are Chinese pear, Japanese pear, Sand, Nashi, and apple pear.

2 **heads Napa cabbage, quartered**

Basic Brine, for soaking (page 92)

2 **daikon radishes, peeled and sliced into matchsticks**

1 **Asian pear, peeled and sliced into matchsticks**

5 **carrots, peeled and sliced into matchsticks**

5 **or 6 scallions, sliced**

2 **inch (5 cm)-long piece fresh ginger, peeled and minced**

1 **head garlic, or 12 medium cloves garlic, chopped**

¼ **cup (60 ml) fish sauce**

½ **cup (260 g) chili paste, or to taste**

¼ **cup (72 g) fine sea salt**

Wash the cabbage leaves and let them soak overnight in enough brine to cover. Once soaked, discard the soaking liquid.

In a large bowl, combine the cabbage with the radishes, pear, carrots, scallions, ginger, garlic, fish sauce, and chili paste. Add the salt to the mixture and combine well. Place the salted mixture, handful by handful, into a large fermentation jar or crock, pounding vigorously after each addition. Liquid will seep from the vegetables. The extracted water should cover the vegetables entirely. If not, add brine to cover. Be sure the level of the liquid stays 1 inch (2.5 cm) below the jar rim to allow for expansion. Press the vegetables down and keep them under the brine by placing a plate or a lid on top, weighted down by a clean rock or resealable plastic bag filled with water.

Leave the fermentation jar in a warm, dark spot in your kitchen to ferment for 5 to 7 days. Check on it periodically to ensure that the brine covers the vegetables. If fruit flies become a problem, cover the jar with a clean towel. It is ready when you are satisfied with the taste. Screw the lid on tightly and transfer it to a cool storage area such as your pantry, basement, or root cellar, where it will continue to ferment. Keeps indefinitely.

Yield: 1 quart (946 ml)

Note You can wake up your morning by adding this kimchi to scrambled eggs, or top it over steamed or fried rice. It's also great in a wrap with mixed greens and meats.

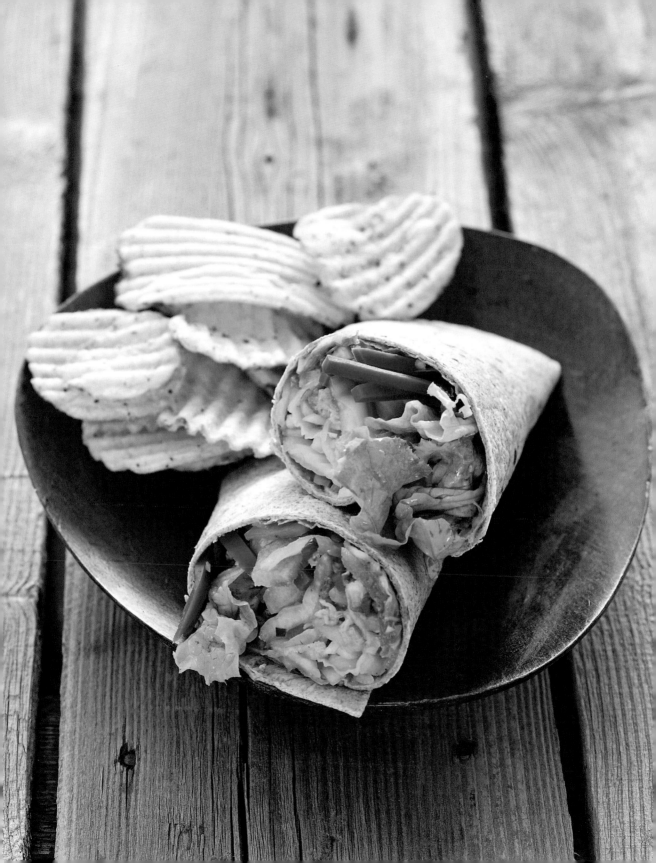

Ginger-Carrot Kraut

Carrots have few rivals when it comes to beta-carotene. A mere ½ cup (40 g) packs a walloping four times the RDA of vitamin A in the form of protective beta-carotene. Fermenting them increases this number substantially.

1 **pound (455 g) carrots, grated**

1 **tablespoon (6 g) peeled, minced fresh ginger**

¼ **cup (60 ml) Easy Whey (page 92)**

1 **quart (946 ml) Basic Brine (page 92)**

Pack the grated carrots into a fermenting jar or crock, then add the ginger. Pour in the whey and brine until the carrots are just covered. Place a smaller jar filled with water (as the weight) on top of the carrots inside the crock.

Let the vegetables ferment for 3 to 5 days in a warm, dark place. Check the carrots every few days, scraping off any mold that forms on the surface, and pressing down on the weight to submerge the carrots in the brine. If fruit flies become a problem, cover the crock with a clean towel. Start tasting the carrots after a few days. They will develop a pleasant, pungent taste but should also maintain some crispness. When satisfied with the taste and texture, screw a lid on the jar tightly and refrigerate. The kraut will keep for several months.

Yield: 1 quart (568 g)

With carrots, you get vitamin A and a host of powerful health benefits. The high level of beta-carotene acts as an antioxidant and is converted into vitamin A in the liver. Beta-carotene has proven effective against macular degeneration and cataracts and even has anticancer and antiaging properties.

Note Ginger is known to have natural analgesic and sedative properties and is a wonderful aid for dyspepsia or stomach ailments. Oranges contain phytonutrients, hesperidin, and polyphenols, which have been shown to lower high blood pressure and cholesterol, and reduce inflammation. Use this relish to add a special tang to baked or grilled meats and fish.

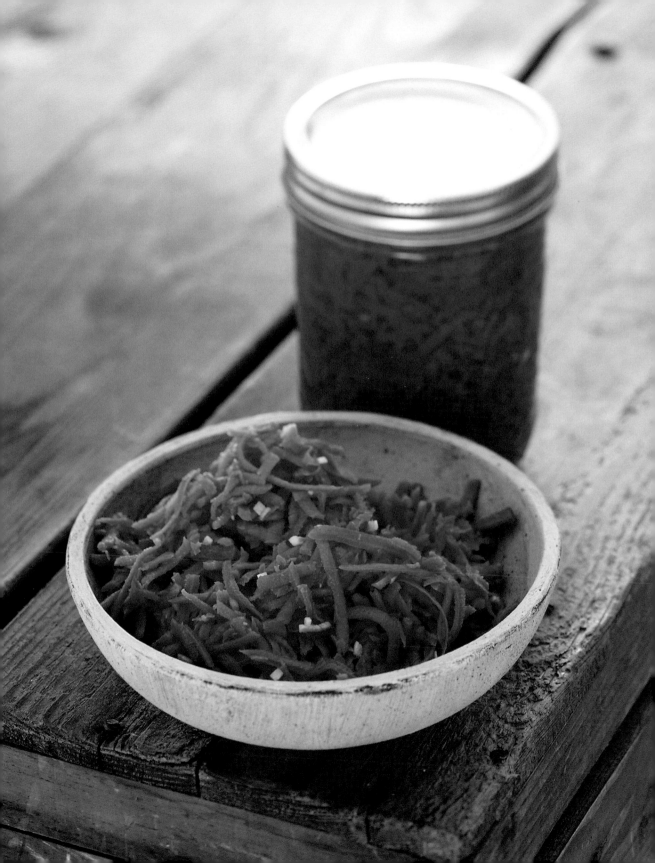

A Peck of Pickled Lacto-Fermented Peppers

Along with its vitamin C and antioxidants, the spicy, pungent, and fiery flavor of pickled jalapeños is enhanced when fermented. A little bit goes a long way with this medicinal beauty.

1 pound (455 g) fresh jalapeño peppers, washed and sliced into ¼-inch (6-mm) rings (seeds removed)

½ red onion, sliced

3 or 4 cloves garlic

¼ cup (60 ml) Easy Whey (page 92)

1 cup (235 ml) Basic Brine (page 92)

Place the peppers, onion, and garlic into your fermenting jar and gently but firmly press down to pack them in. Pour the whey and brine over the vegetables to cover. Be sure the level of the liquid stays 1 inch (2.5 cm) below the jar rim to allow for expansion. Place a lid tightly on the jar and allow to ferment at room temperature until the jalapeños change color from deep green to an olive green. This usually takes 4 to 6 days, depending on the temperature of your kitchen. Transfer to the refrigerator.

Yield: 1 quart (946 ml)

The health-benefiting alkaloid compound, capsaicin—the chemical that makes chile peppers hot—is known to have antibacterial, anticarcinogenic, and cholesterol-lowering properties. It's also known to inhibit a key neuropeptide, Substance P, that is the key brain-pain transmitter, meaning it can provide relief for migraines and sinus pain. Capsaicin is also used in the preparation of ointments, rubs, and tinctures for its pain-relieving properties.

Note In addition to probiotics, whey is high in amino acids, electrolytes, and B-complex vitamins.

Cleansing Beets with Ginger and Grapefruit

Vibrant, crunchy, and tangy, beets are just loaded with nutrients. Because beets have the highest sugar content of all vegetables, they pair nicely with the tart flavor of grapefruit and the warming ginger. You can't go wrong with this delicious digestive aid that's loaded with color.

6 medium (or 4 large) tender young beets, trimmed and chopped or shredded, with peels left on

1 inch (2.5 cm)-long piece fresh ginger, peeled and cut into matchsticks

Zest of ½ small to medium grapefruit, or 1 large orange

⅛ teaspoon ground cloves

Seeds from 2 cardamom pods (optional)

½ cup (120 ml) Easy Whey (page 92)

Basic Brine, as needed (page 92)

2 cinnamon sticks

In a medium bowl, combine the beets, ginger, grapefruit zest, cloves, and cardamom seeds. Place this mixture into a wide-mouth fermenting jar. Cover the beets with the whey, adding as much brine as needed, to completely submerge the mixture. Add the cinnamon sticks. Be sure the level of the liquid stays 1 inch (2.5 cm) below the jar rim. Cover the jar tightly with a lid or an airlock and allow to ferment in a dark, cool spot at room temperature for 3 to 5 days. Transfer the jar to the refrigerator, where the beets will continue to ferment at a slower rate. This will keep for several months.

Yield: About 1 quart (946 ml)

Note *Enjoy with salads or meat dishes, or use these beets to make borscht— a classic Russian soup that's eaten cold.*

Antioxidant-Rich Asparagus Spears

Nothing heralds the onset of spring like crisp, fresh asparagus. Although these fleshy spears are valued for their tender texture and succulent taste, asparagus also packs a lot of nutritional value. You'll love the aroma and flavors in this antioxidant-rich blend teeming with probiotics.

½ **teaspoon black peppercorns**

¼ **teaspoon celery seed**

½ **teaspoon coriander seeds**

2 **cloves garlic, thinly sliced (optional)**

Approximately 40 young asparagus stalks, cut in half, bottom ends trimmed off

¼ **whole lemon**

¼ **cup (60 ml) Easy Whey (page 92)**

2 **cups (475 ml) Basic Brine (page 92), plus more as needed**

In a 1-quart (946-ml) fermenting jar, combine the peppercorns, celery seed, coriander seeds, and garlic.

Pack the asparagus stalks upright in the jar, leaving 1 inch (2.5 cm) free at the top. Push the lemon wedge in between the asparagus spears. Pour the whey into the jar, then pour the brine on top. Be sure the level of the liquid stays 1 inch (2.5 cm) below the jar rim to allow for expansion. Cover the jar tightly with a lid or an airlock, and allow to ferment in a dark spot at room temperature for 2 to 3 days. Transfer the jar to the refrigerator, where the asparagus will continue to ferment at a slower rate.

Yield: 1 quart (700 g)

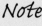 *Asparagus is loaded with vitamins A, C, E, and K, along with minerals such as folate, iron, and potassium. They're high in fiber, too, making them an attractive prebiotic food.*

Note *These are delicious served with poached eggs for breakfast. Or serve over a green garden salad or rice pilaf.*

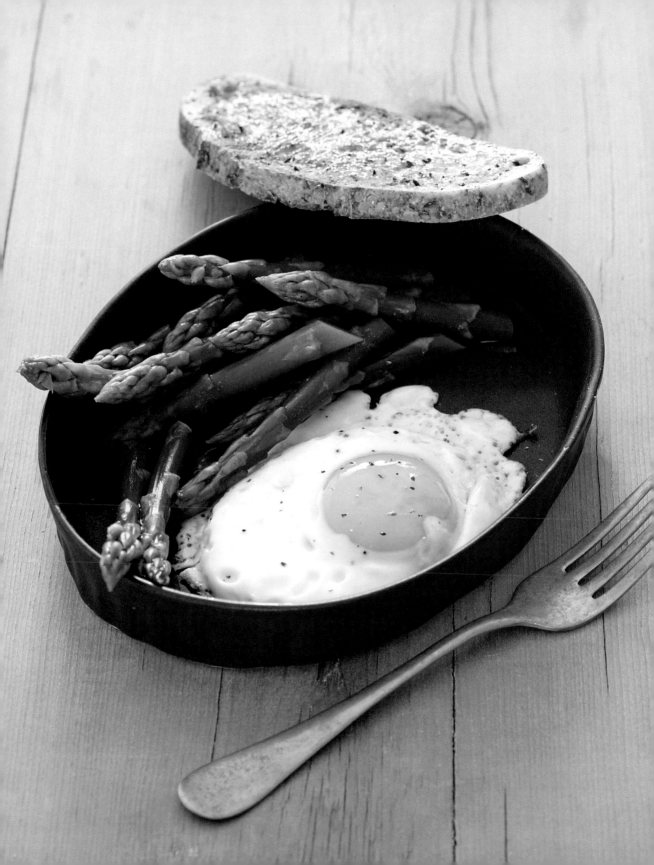

Enzyme-Rich Tomatillo and Mint Salsa

Loaded with enzymes, tomatillos are a treasure when it comes to their antioxidants. The high enzyme content actually serves to enhance the activity of the antioxidants. Naturally, their nutrients and bioavailability are enhanced through fermentation.

2 **pounds (1 kg) tomatillos, chopped**

1 **large red onion, chopped**

6 **cloves garlic, peeled and chopped**

3 **chile peppers, seeded and chopped**

½ **cup (8 g) cilantro, coarsely chopped**

¼ **cup (24 g) fresh mint, coarsely chopped**

Juice of 1 lemon or lime

½ **cup (120 ml) Easy Whey (page 92)**

Dash of cayenne pepper

½ **teaspoon ground cumin**

2 **teaspoons fine sea salt**

Place the tomatillos, onion, garlic, chile peppers, cilantro, and mint into the bowl of a food processor and process until smooth. Transfer to a large bowl and add the lemon or lime juice, whey, cayenne, cumin, and salt, and combine well. Pour into a wide-mouth fermenting jar and cap tightly. Leave to ferment at room temperature for 3 to 5 days. Check on it periodically to ensure that the brine still covers the vegetables. Transfer to the refrigerator, where the salsa will keep for up to 4 weeks, and the flavor will intensify.

Yield: About 1 quart (946 ml)

Tomatillos are especially rich in lycopene, which plays a special role in bone and cardiovascular health.

Note Tomatillos are sometimes called "green tomatoes." They should not, however, be confused with green, unripe tomatoes, which are in the same family but of a different genus. Choose your tomatillos by a combination of flavor, texture, and appearance.

You can get the benefits of fermented salsa by adding Easy Whey (page 92) to store-bought salsa. Experiment with fermenting ketchup, barbecue sauce, and pasta sauce in the same way.

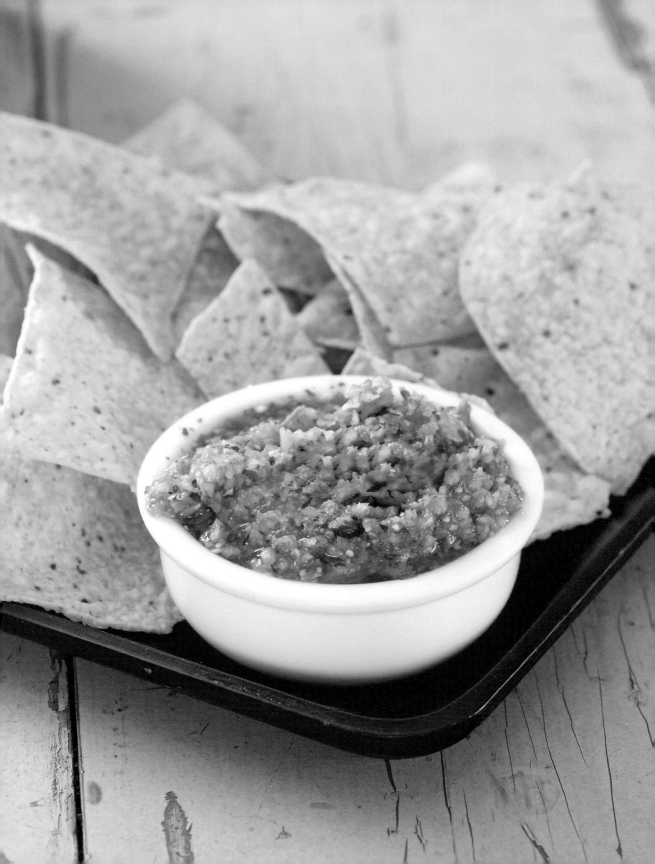

Digestive Pickled Radishes with Ginger and Apple

Crisp, bright, and tangy, fermented radishes are especially good for aiding digestion. The addition of cumin and coriander increases their digestive capabilities, while the apple adds even more fiber and flavor. Loaded with probiotics, this is wonderfully delicious eaten atop summer salads.

About 30 radishes, trimmed and cut into slices or quarters

3 cloves garlic, minced

1 large (or 2 small) red onions, thinly sliced

1 inch (2.5 cm)-long piece fresh ginger, cut into ¼-inch (6-mm) slices

1 medium apple, peeled, cored, and chopped

½ teaspoon cumin seeds

½ teaspoon coriander

½ small chile pepper, chopped (optional)

¼ cup (60 ml) Easy Whey (page 92)

1 cup (235 ml) Basic Brine, plus more as needed (page 92)

Combine the radishes, garlic, onion, ginger, apple, cumin seeds, coriander, and chile pepper in a large bowl. Transfer them to a 1-quart (946-ml) fermenting jar or crock, and add the whey. Cover all ingredients with the brine. Be sure the level of the liquid stays 1 inch (2.5 cm) below the jar rim to allow for expansion. Gently press the ingredients down and cap tightly.

Leave to ferment at room temperature for 3 to 5 days, checking on it periodically to ensure that the brine still covers the vegetables. Transfer to the refrigerator. Will keep refrigerated for several months.

Yield: About 1 quart (946 ml)

Radish leaves contain almost six times the amount of vitamin C as their roots and are a good source of calcium and potassium.

Note The radish belongs to the Brassicaceae family.
Radish is also known as "daikon" in some parts of the world.

Stress-Less Gazpacho

A summertime staple, gazpacho is notable for its piquant flavor, hearty texture, and easy preparation. Nutritionally, it is loaded with lycopene antioxidants, which are absorbed more easily by the addition of olive oil. Fermenting gazpacho with whey increases its already high vitamin C and phytochemical content. A nutrition study done on volunteers who ate gazpacho every day for two weeks showed significant increase in blood levels of vitamin C and a decrease in key stress molecules.

4 **medium tomatoes, peeled and roughly chopped**

1 **medium cucumber, roughly chopped**

1 **yellow or red bell pepper, roughly chopped**

1 **red or sweet onion, roughly chopped**

2 **cloves garlic, minced**

½ **cup (30 g) chopped fresh parsley**

2 **tablespoons (2 g) chopped cilantro**

1 **chile pepper, seeded and chopped**

1 **cup (235 ml) tomato or vegetable juice**

½ **cup (120 ml) filtered water**

  Juice of 1 lime

1 **tablespoon (15 ml) extra-virgin olive oil**

3 **tablespoons (45 ml) Easy Whey (page 92)**

1 **teaspoon fine sea salt**

  Freshly ground black pepper

Place the tomatoes, cucumber, bell pepper, onion, garlic, parsley, cilantro, and chile pepper into the container of a blender and blend until chunky. Pour half the mixture into a large bowl. Add the tomato juice, water, lime juice, olive oil, and whey to the remaining mixture in the blender and blend until smooth. Transfer the blended ingredients to the bowl, and season with salt and pepper. Cover the bowl and refrigerate for 1 to 2 days. Serve cold.

Yield: About 1½ quarts (1420 ml)

Garlic Dill Pickles Delight

Loaded with beneficial bacteria, sour pickles are crunchy and tangy, and the flavor gets better with time. This version adds garlic, mustard, and dill to enhance flavor even more. The fermentation of garlic more than doubles the amount of antioxidants and produces a rich, savory flavor.

8 to 10 unwaxed or organic pickling cucumbers

1 tablespoon (4 g) chopped fresh dill

8 to 10 cloves garlic, peeled

1 tablespoon (11 g) mustard seeds

1 tablespoon (18 g) fine sea salt

¼ cup (60 ml) Easy Whey (page 92)

1½ cups (355 ml) Basic Brine (page 92)

Wash the cucumbers well. Divide them in half and place them in two 2-quart (2-L) fermenting jars. Combine the dill, garlic, and mustard seeds in a small bowl. Divide the mixture evenly between the two jars and pour it over the cucumbers, adding salt as you go. Add the whey and then the brine evenly between each jar, covering the cucumbers completely so they are submerged 1 inch (2.5 cm) below the liquid. Cover the jars tightly with lids and let sit at room temperature for 5 to 10 days. Taste the cucumbers occasionally during the process to see if they are done. When you are satisfied with the taste, transfer the jars to the refrigerator, where they will keep for several months.

Yield: About 2 quarts (2 L)

Cucumbers have diuretic properties because of their high water and potassium content, which aids in reducing both weight and high blood pressure.

Note Enjoy the gustatory adventure and tantalizing taste of these refreshing pickles as an accompaniment to any meat, fish, salad, or rice dish.

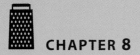

CHAPTER 8

Fruits

One of the great things about fermenting fruits is that their naturally sweet taste nicely complements the sour taste created through lacto-fermentation. You can use many of these chutneys and jams as an accompaniment to add richness and flavor to your fish, chicken, and beef dishes. You will also be giving your digestive system a huge boost.

Fermented Mango, Cinnamon, and Peach Chutney

The king of exotic fruits, mangos—as well as peaches—not only taste delicious, but they are also rich in nutrients and prebiotic dietary fiber. Best of all, when fermented, both fruits offer a sweet and tart treat that won't make you crave sugar.

8 to 10 peaches, peeled, cored, and quartered

4 ripe mangos, peeled, seeded, and coarsely chopped

1 cup (145 g) raisins

2 cups (200 g) pecans, chopped

2 teaspoons fine sea salt

Juice of 4 lemons

¼ cup (32 g) grated fresh ginger

2 chile peppers, seeded and chopped

2 tablespoons (14 g) ground cinnamon

¼ cup (60 ml) Easy Whey (page 92)

Basic Brine (page 92), as needed

In a large bowl, combine the peaches, mangos, raisins, pecans, salt, lemon juice, ginger, chile peppers, and cinnamon. Place the mixture into a fermentation jar and tamp it down until it's no more than 1 inch (2.5 cm) below the jar rim to allow for expansion. Pour in the whey. Allow the extracted juices and whey to cover the mixture then add brine as needed. Keep the contents 1 inch (2.5 cm) below the rim to allow for expansion. Press the fruit mixture, down into the jar and keep it under the brine by placing a plate or a lid on top, weighted down by a clean rock or resealable plastic bag filled with water. Cover with a clean cloth to keep out fruit flies.

Place the fermentation jar in a dark spot in your kitchen at room temperature. Allow the chutney to ferment for 2 to 4 days. Check on it periodically to ensure that the brine covers the mixture and to remove any mold that may form on the surface. Taste the chutney during the fermentation process, and when you are satisfied with the taste, cap it, and transfer it to the refrigerator.

Yield: About 1 quart (946 ml)

Notes *This dish is perfect for an afternoon snack, an evening dessert, or as an accompaniment to beef, pork, or fish. To peel peaches, drop the quarters into a pot of boiling water for only 5 to 10 seconds, then plunge into an ice water bath.*

Amino acids, vitamins C and E, calcium, iron, magnesium, and potassium are among the medicinal compounds in mangos and peaches. Mango peels are also rich in phytonutrients, such as carotenoids. You can ferment the peels, then place then in a food dehydrator to make fruit leather.

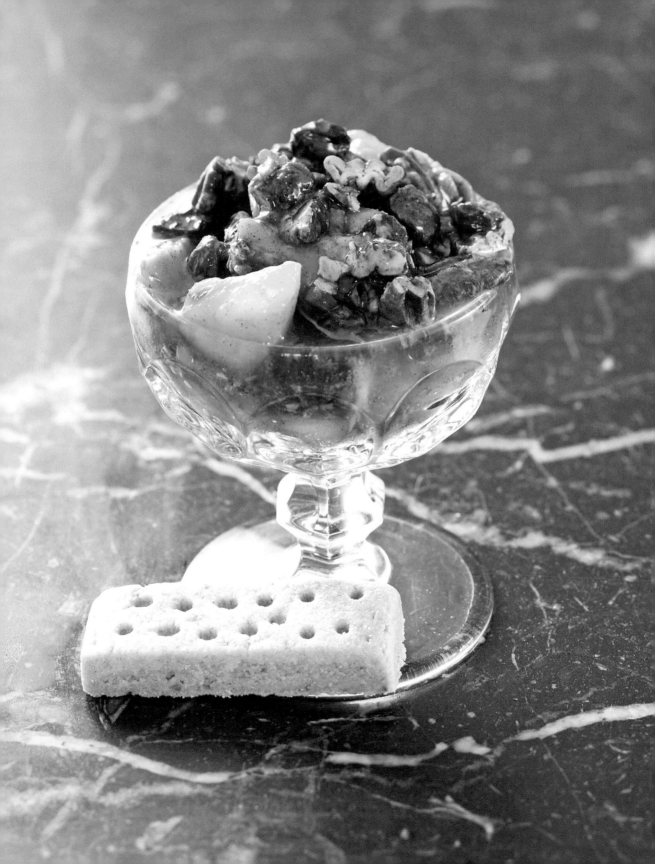

Plum Yum Prune Sauce

Wonderfully delicious and juicy, plums and prunes contain more than double the antioxidants, especially vitamin C, than most other fruits; the amount of antioxidants is, of course, enhanced through fermentation. High in prebiotic fiber, prunes and plums are good for digestion and speed up your metabolism.

3 to 4 plums, halved and pitted

1   cup (175 g) pitted prunes

¼ cup (85 g) unrefined sweetener (rapadura, raw honey, or maple syrup)

1   teaspoon fine sea salt

¼ cup (60 ml) Easy Whey (page 92)

Place the plums, prunes, sweetener, salt, and whey in a food processor bowl and process until smooth. Transfer the mixture to a wide-mouth quart jar or crock, leaving 1 inch (2.5 mm) free below the jar rim to allow for expansion. Cover tightly with a lid or airlock. Leave at room temperature for 2 to 3 days, then transfer to the refrigerator. The sauce will keep for a few weeks.

Yield: 1 quart (946 ml)

Enzyme-Potent Papaya-Kombucha Smoothie ▶

This luscious smoothie contains all the beneficial microorganisms of kombucha, plus a high level of digestive enzymes from papaya. Kombucha is probiotic-rich living food that is made from tea and can be flavored with your favorite fruits, spices, and other ingredients (see page 56).

2½ cups (440 g) diced papaya

1   teaspoon ground cinnamon

1   tablespoon (20 g) locally harvested raw honey

1½ cups (355 ml) kombucha tea

Place the papaya, cinnamon, and honey into the container of a blender and process until all the fruit has been puréed. Add the kombucha and blend until well mixed.

Yield: 1 quart (946 ml)

Note A kombucha culture starter is called a SCOBY. It stands for symbiotic culture of bacteria and yeast.

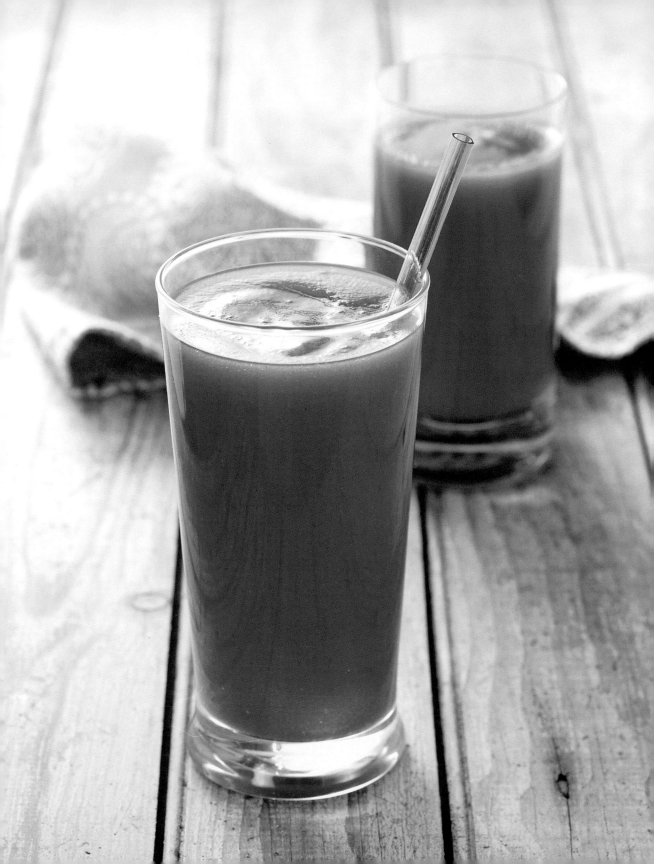

Lacto-Fermented Lemons or Limes

Enjoy the sour taste of these preserved lemons or limes, which are alkalinizing to the stomach and promote healthy digestion. They are rich in beneficial bacteria and outstanding in their vitamin C, flavonoids, and enzyme content.

Juice of 3 lemons

½ cup (144 g) fine sea salt

1 tablespoon (6 g) coriander

7 or 8 organic lemons or limes, ends trimmed

1 cinnamon stick

1 chile pepper

2 bay leaves

Combine the lemon juice with the salt and coriander. Roll the whole lemons or limes on a kitchen countertop to soften; slice them crosswise into quarters, stopping ½ inch (13 mm) from the bottom, so the sections remain connected. Sprinkle the interior of the fruit with half the lemon juice mixture. Layer the lemons or limes into a wide-mouth fermenting jar no higher than the shoulder of the jar. Pour the remaining lemon juice mixture over the lemons until juice is ½ inch (13 mm) above them. Add filtered water, if necessary. Add the cinnamon stick, chile pepper, and bay leaves. Using a wooden spoon or dowel, press down on the fruit to soften the rinds and to allow the lemons or limes to release their juices, which will combine with the salt to create a brine. Secure with a lid or an airlock and ferment at room temperature for 30 days, checking them every few days to ensure brine level. Then refrigerate. Lemons and limes can be kept for 1 year, possibly longer.

Yield: 7 or 8 lemons or limes

Apple Blackberry Kraut Crunch ▶

Combining blackberries and apples with cabbage adds a delicious sweet flavor and tons more nutrients. This kraut is loaded with prebiotics, probiotics, and antioxidants, and the walnuts increase its omega-3s while giving a crunchy, fiber-filled texture.

½ small cabbage, shredded

1 teaspoon fine sea salt

1 apple, peeled, cored, and finely chopped

Juice of 1 orange (include some pulp)

1 cup (120 g) chopped walnuts

½ cup (75 g) blackberries

1 teaspoon broken pieces of cinnamon sticks

¼ cup (60 ml) Easy Whey (page 92)

Place the cabbage in a bowl and sprinkle with the salt. Add the apple, orange juice, walnuts, blackberries, and cinnamon, and mix well. Firmly pack the mixture into a wide-mouth 1-quart (946-ml) jar. Pour in the whey; add water, if necessary, to cover the mixture completely. Be sure the level of the liquid stays 1 inch (2.5 cm) below the jar rim to allow for expansion. Seal the jar tightly with a lid or an airlock. Leave at room temperature for 5 to 6 days, then refrigerate. This will keep for a few weeks.

Yield: 1 quart (946 ml)

> *Note* Serve alongside salads or use it to top yogurt.

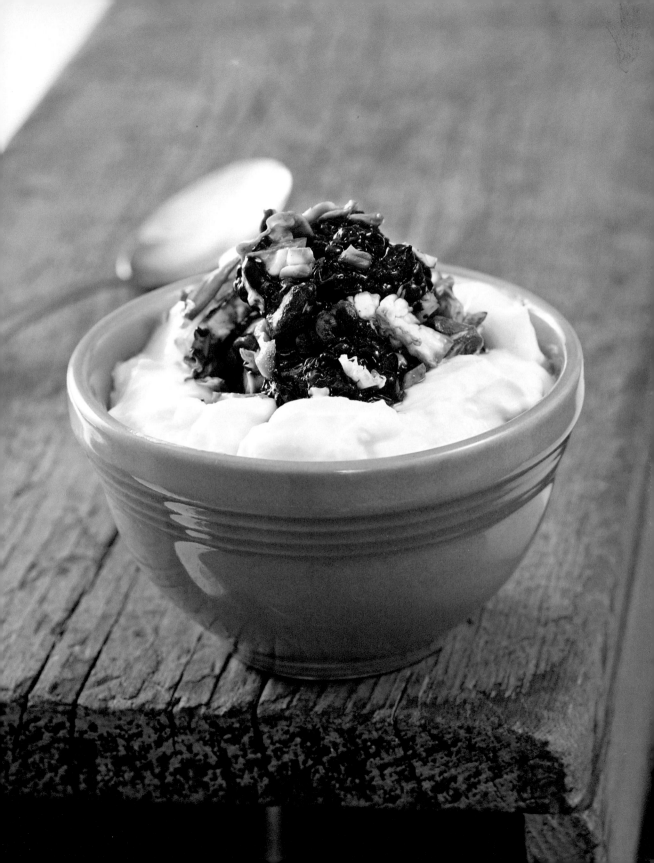

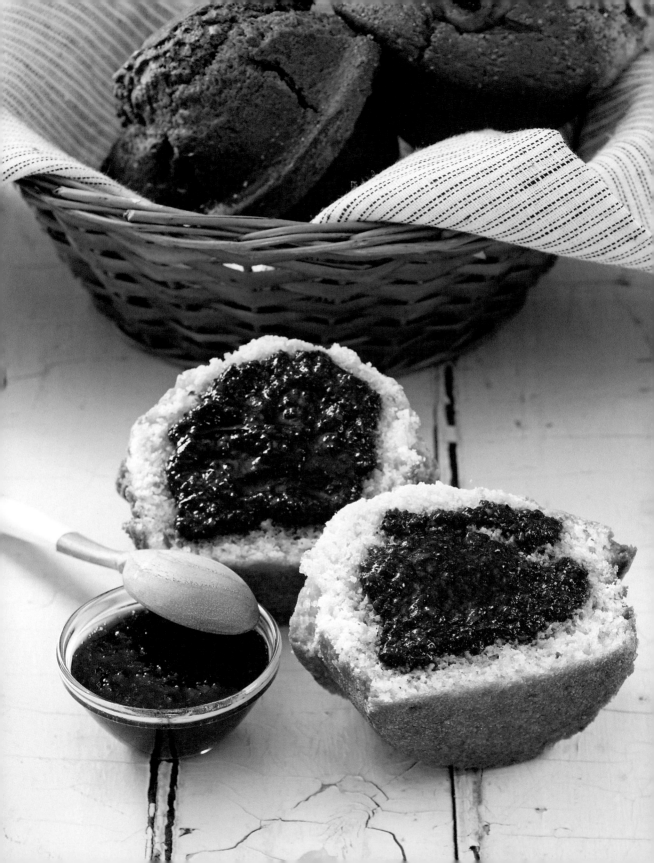

Probiotic Berry-Good-for-You Jam

There's nothing better than the tangy taste of homemade jam at breakfast or for a sweet treat, and fermenting it only adds to the guiltless pleasure. This jam is also a great way to introduce the kids to fermented foods; top it over toast, waffles, or pancakes.

3 cups (435 g) fresh berries (cherry, blackberry, raspberry, blueberry), or 2 to 3 cups (260–390 g) unsulfured dried fruit (apricots, figs, raisins, dates, pineapple, papaya, cranberry)

¼ cup plus 2 tablespoons (90 ml) Easy Whey (page 92), divided

2 teaspoons fine sea salt

2 teaspoons Pomona's universal pectin (available at health food stores)

¼ cup (60 ml) natural sweetener (rapadura, raw honey, maple syrup), plus more, as desired

If using fresh fruit: Place the fruit in a bowl and add the ¼ cup (60 ml) whey, salt, pectin, and sweetener; mash everything together. If using dried fruit: Place the fruit in a bowl and cover with hot, filtered water. Allow the fruit to soak for 20 minutes, or until hydrated. Drain the fruit, then transfer to the bowl of a food processor and add the ¼ cup (60 ml) whey, salt, pectin, and sweetener. Pulse once or twice to combine, then process until it forms a paste.

Transfer the fresh fruit mixture or dried fruit mixture to a fermenting jar. Pour the remaining 2 tablespoons (30 ml) whey over the fruit. Set the jar in a dark place and allow it to ferment for 2 to 3 days at room temperature.

Transfer the fruit to the bowl of a food processor and add more sweetener to taste; process until smooth. Serve immediately or transfer to a jar and refrigerate. Should keep for up to 2 months in the refrigerator.

Yield: About 1 pint (473 ml)

Berries are packed with antioxidants and flavonoids. A diet rich in berries reduces inflammation, which prevents cellular damage and improves blood pressure and HDL ("good") cholesterol levels.

Apple, Ginger, and Mint Chutney with a Kick

Fiber-rich apples are loaded with enzymes and are a good source of polyphenols, which function as antioxidants. Paired with the ginger, this chutney makes an amazing digestive aid and blood sugar balancer. The addition of fresh mint and chiles offers a gentle kick.

4 to 6 ripe apples, peeled, cored, and chopped

1 inch (2.5 cm)-long piece fresh ginger, peeled and minced

1 cup (96 g) fresh mint leaves, finely minced

2 chile peppers, seeded and minced

¼ cup plus 2 tablespoons (90 ml) Easy Whey (page 92), divided

Place the apples, ginger, mint, and chile peppers in the bowl of a food processor and process until smooth. Stir in the ¼ cup (60 ml) whey. Spoon the chutney mixture into a wide-mouth fermentation jar in batches and mash with a wooden spoon until the apples release their juice. Continue spooning the chutney into the jar, mashing it with a spoon, until all the mixture is in the jar and the liquid covers the apple solids. Spoon the remaining 2 tablespoons (30 ml) whey over the chutney. Be sure the level of the liquid stays 1 inch (2.5 cm) below the jar rim to allow for expansion. Cover it loosely with a towel to keep out any fruit flies. Allow the chutney to ferment in a dark spot at room temperature for 2 to 3 days. Screw a lid on tightly and refrigerate. This should keep for several weeks.

Yield: About 1 quart (946 ml)

Digestive Pineapple Chutney ▶

This chutney is sweet, tart, and juicy, and loaded with enzymes to keep the digestive tract healthy. Kids love it, too.

1 small ripe pineapple, peeled, cored, and chopped

1 cup (16 g) finely minced cilantro

1 inch (2.5 cm)-long piece fresh ginger, peeled and minced

2 chile peppers, seeded, if desired, and minced

¼ cup (60 ml) Easy Whey (page 92)

In the bowl of a food processor, combine the pineapple, cilantro, ginger, and chile peppers until the pineapple is finely chopped and ingredients are well mixed. Stir in the whey. Transfer the ingredients to a fermenting jar and mash with a wooden spoon until the pineapple releases its juice. Allow liquid to cover the contents, leaving 1 to 2 inches (2.5–5 cm) from the top of the jar for the pineapple to expand as it ferments. Cover with a towel or loose-fitting lid (or use an airlock). Let sit for 2 to 3 days at room temperature; cap tightly and refrigerate. This will keep for up to 2 months.

Yield: 1 quart (946 ml)

> *Note* Pineapple contains one of the most important enzymes, bromelain, which helps in the digestion of protein. Pineapples can also greatly alleviate the pain of arthritis due to their anti-inflammatory properties.

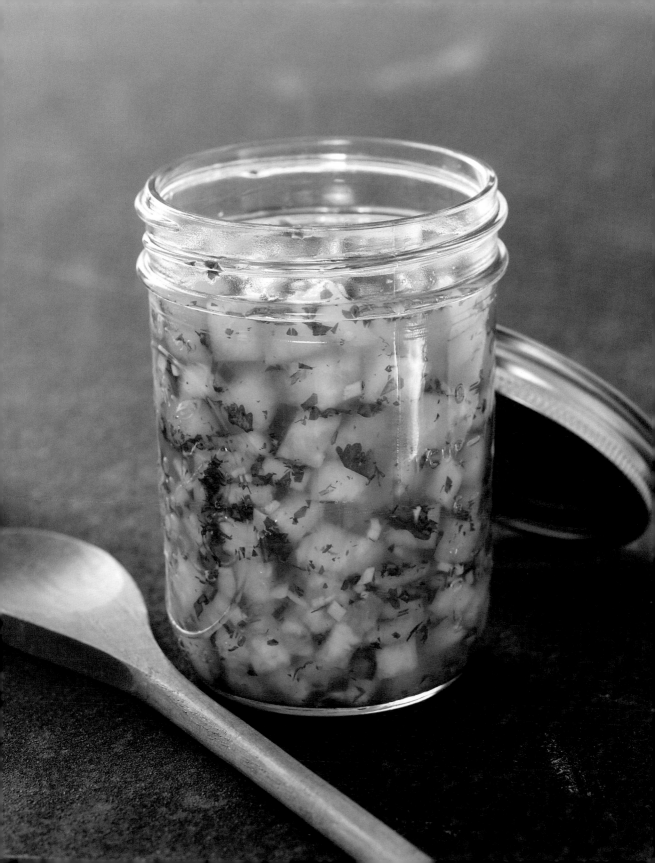

Fiber-Filled Fig and Apricot Honey Butter

Apart from their succulent flesh and fabulous flavor, figs are filled with prebiotic fiber to promote healthy microflora and strengthen the immune system. Figs grow on the Ficus tree, which is a member of the Moraceae, or mulberry, family. After Turkey and Greece, California ranks third in the world in production of figs. Black mission figs are the highest in antioxidants. Apricots are well known for their high content of fiber, vitamins, minerals, and antioxidants. They are a great source of beta-carotene, giving you nearly 50 percent of your daily value of vitamin A. Together, figs and apricots pack a powerful nutritious punch.

1 **cup (150 g) dried or fresh figs**

1 **cup (165 g) dried or fresh apricots, pitted**

¼ **cup plus 1 tablespoon (75 ml) Easy Whey (page 92), divided**

2 **tablespoons (40 g) locally harvested raw honey**

¼ **teaspoon crushed cloves**

Dash of cayenne pepper (optional)

If using dried fruit: Place the fruit in a bowl and cover with hot filtered water for 15 to 20 minutes, until hydrated. Drain the fruit and transfer it to the bowl of a food processor. If using fresh fruit: Roughly chop, then transfer it to the bowl of a food processor.

Add the ¼ cup (60 ml) whey and pulse the dried or fresh fruit mixture once or twice to combine, then process until the fruit forms a paste (for dried) or is well blended (for fresh). Transfer to a fermenting jar and cover with the remaining 1 tablespoon (15 ml) whey, if needed. Cap the jar and let it sit out to ferment for 2 to 3 days at room temperature.

Transfer the contents of the jar to the bowl of a food processor and add the honey, cloves, and cayenne. Process until smooth. Serve immediately, or transfer to a screw-top jar and refrigerate. Butter should keep up for to 2 months in the refrigerator.

Yield: 2 cups (473 ml)

Note Use this delicious mix to top yogurt or pancakes, or on sourdough toast (see page 135)

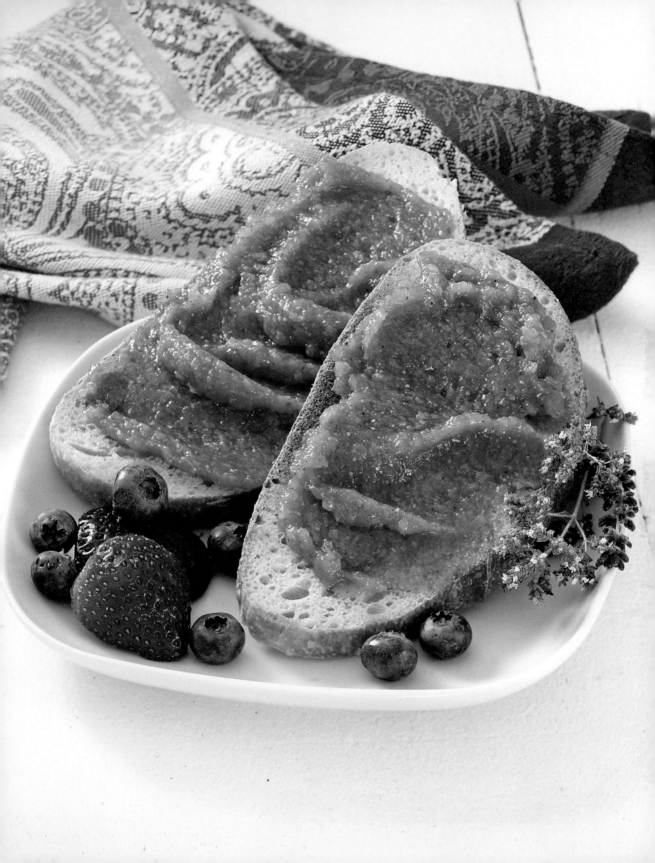

Tropical Coconut, Mango, and Mint Chutney

Loaded with enzymes, the combination of mango and coconut creates a delicious tropical punch to this summer chutney.

3 cups (525 g) tightly packed, coarsely chopped, peeled mangos

⅛ teaspoon ground cloves

½ cup (40 g) unsweetened shredded coconut

1 tablespoon (6 g) chopped fresh mint leaves, or 1 teaspoon dried

2 tablespoons (40 g) unrefined sweetener (rapadura, raw honey, maple syrup)

¼ cup (60 ml) Easy Whey (page 92)

1 teaspoon fine sea salt

In a medium-size mixing bowl, combine the mangos, cloves, coconut, mint, sweetener, whey, and salt. Transfer the mixture to a half-gallon (2-L) jar or crock. Pack down well to at least 1 to 2 inches (2.5–5 cm) below the rim of the container. Seal the jar tightly with a lid or an airlock. Leave the jar on the kitchen counter for 2 to 3 days, then refrigerate. Chutney will keep for a few weeks.

Yield: 1 pint (475 ml)

The nutrients present in mango improve digestion and are known to boost libido. And there's no end to the wide array of nutritional benefits derived from coconuts. They are well known for their amazing ability to fight harmful bacteria and ward off countless infections.

Note Try different fruits, such as apples or cherries, to create a variety of flavors.

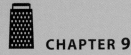

CHAPTER 9

Grains and Beans

Apart from neutralizing the phytic acid and other anti-nutrients in grains and beans, soaking and fermenting them also breaks down gluten, sugars, and other difficult-to-digest elements. You can use dried beans in these recipes, but it's also okay to substitute canned beans if that's all you have. Just remember to soak canned beans first, though, before fermenting them because they usually are not soaked before canning, leaving the enzyme inhibitors in the beans.

Enzyme-Powered Natto Sushi Rolls

If you're feeling daring, this dish is well worth your efforts, both for your body and for your taste buds. Natto is little more than cooked soybeans that have been fermented, which makes them easy to digest, and its friendly microflora helps strengthen immunity. This Japanese staple has a sticky texture and pungent taste that may be new to you. Toasted nori, which is edible seaweed that comes in sheets, is available in health food stores and some supermarkets. Though not essential, sushi rolling mats simplify this procedure and can be found online and in many kitchen retail stores.

For the natto:

2 **cups (400 g) dried soybeans**

7 **cups (1645 ml) filtered water, divided**

1 **teaspoon natto bacteria starter culture (see Resources)**

½ **teaspoon fine sea salt**

½ **teaspoon brown sugar**

For the sushi rolls:

4 **sheets toasted nori**

2 **cups (330 g) Sprouted Enzymatic Brown Rice (page 130)**

½ **cup (86 g) natto**

3 **scallions, sliced into strips**

To make the natto: Rinse the soybeans, then soak them in 4 cups (940 ml) filtered water in a large bowl for 24 hours at room temperature. The soybeans will double in size. Drain the beans in a colander and place the colander directly into a pressure cooker. Pour the remaining 3 cups (705 ml) filtered water into the pressure cooker and secure the lid. Set over high heat for 15 minutes, then allow to cool for 2 hours.

Preheat the oven to 100°F (38°C), or prepare a food dehydrator.

Open the pressure cooker and sprinkle the soybeans with the natto bacteria starter culture, salt, and brown sugar. Stir gently to coat the beans. Transfer the beans to a baking dish and cover with aluminum foil. Place in the oven or food dehydrator and leave undisturbed for 48 hours. (If using the oven, you will need to prop open the oven door about 2 inches [5 cm] to maintain this temperature.)

Remove the beans from the oven or food dehydrator and refrigerate them. They will keep for up to 2 weeks.

To make the sushi rolls: Lay 1 sheet of nori over a bamboo rolling mat. Spoon ½ cup (83 g) rice over the nori and press firmly. Layer with the natto and scallions along the center of the rice and roll up. Slice the roll into 6 pieces. Repeat with the 3 remaining nori sheets. Serve immediately or refrigerate. Delicious with Plum Yum Prune Sauce (page 116)!

Yield: 4 rolls (24 pieces)

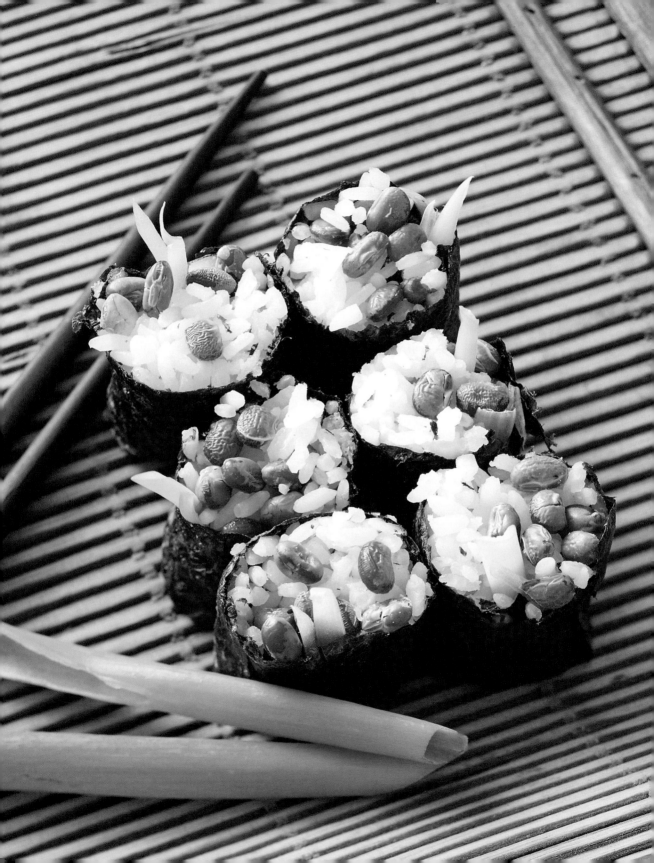

Sprouted Enzymatic Brown Rice

Sprouted rice is higher in nutritional value than non-sprouted rice because the process of germination enhances the bio-availability of enzymes, vitamins, and minerals by neutralizing the phytic acid. Sprouted rice is not only tastier, but it also has more fiber and ten times the amount of essential amino acids as those in non-sprouted rice. You get plenty of benefits from a few minutes of preparation and a few hours of soaking.

- **1½ cups (285 g) whole-grain, unprocessed brown rice**
- **3 cups (705 ml) filtered water**
- **1 tablespoon (15 ml) brown rice vinegar**
- **1 tablespoon (13 g) sugar**
- **2 teaspoons fine sea salt**

Rinse the rice in a colander under flowing water for 1 to 2 minutes. Place the rice in a mixing bowl or wide-mouth fermenting jar with enough warm water to cover by 2 inches (5 cm). Soak for 12 hours. Pour the rice into a mesh sieve and rinse well. Throw out the rinsing water and rinse the bowl or jar. Pour the rice back into the bowl or jar; cover with a clean towel to allow it to breathe. Place the container in a cool, dark place.

Stir the rice well with a wooden spoon twice a day for 2 days. The rice will begin to germinate. Rinse the rice one last time, then toss onto a mesh drying rack or something similar that allows for drainage. Store the rice in the refrigerator for 1 to 2 weeks.

Cook the rice as you normally would: Bring the 3 cups (705 ml) filtered water to a boil, add the rice, and simmer, covered, until done. (Sprouted rice cooks much more quickly than non-sprouted.) As the rice cooks, whisk together the vinegar, sugar, and salt does in a bowl until well combined, and then add it to the cooked rice.

Yield: About 3 cups (495 g)

Note Any time you soak rice for longer than 12 hours, you will need to change the water; just drain and refill with fresh water to continue soaking. Don't let the germinated "tails" grow more than ⅛ inch (3 mm) long, or they'll become bitter. Sprout only as much rice as you can eat within 1 to 2 weeks; after that, it turns bitter. As a general rule, ⅔ cup (127 g) of dried rice will sprout to about 1 cup (190 g). Use sprouted rice for side dishes, rice salads, and breakfast grains.

Lacto-Fermented Lentils

Rich in protein, lentils are high in both soluble and insoluble dietary fiber, making them an ideal prebiotic food. Fermenting them greatly enhances their nutritional value and content. They are quick and easy to prepare and readily absorb a variety of flavors from the foods and seasonings they're prepared with.

1 cup (192 g) dried lentils

2 cups (475 ml) warm filtered water

2 tablespoons (30 ml) Easy Whey (page 92) or yogurt

1 tablespoon (15 ml) raw vinegar, or the juice of a small lemon

1 teaspoon fine sea salt

1 tablespoon (6 g) ground coriander

1 tablespoon (7 g) ground cumin

Sift the lentils and pick through them, removing anything that does not look like a lentil. Place them in a bowl and stir; add the filtered water and the whey, and stir again. Add the vinegar or lemon juice. Stir, and cover with a clean cloth. Let soak for 24 hours in a cool place at room temperature, changing the water after 12 hours. Drain and rinse the lentils.

Place the lentils in a medium saucepan over medium-high heat, and add the salt and filtered water to cover by a couple inches. Bring to a boil; cover and reduce the heat to low and simmer, stirring occasionally, about 20 to 30 minutes, or until the lentils are tender. Drain, then season with the coriander and cumin. For a change, you can flavor with oils or other herbs and spices, such as olive oil, ginger, and garlic.

Yield: 2½ cups (425 g)

Lentils are high in folic acid, magnesium, vitamins C and B complex, iron, manganese, potassium, and phosphorus.

Note There are many different types of lentils, which range in color from red, green, and orange to brown and black and can be bought with or without their skins, though it's not necessary to use skinless lentils for fermenting purposes. Add them to soups, salads, or stir-fries, or use them to make Love-Your-Heart Lentil Dal (page 143).

Weight-Reducing
Tempeh Coconut Curry

It doesn't get better than these two amazing functional foods in one dish. Tempeh has been a highly nutritious fermented staple of Indonesia for over two thousand years due to its high protein content, which makes it a wonderful substitute for meat. Coconut milk adds a rich, creamy texture and contains lauric acid, an antiviral, antibacterial, and antifungal agent. Together with the spices and vegetables, this combination of tempeh and coconut milk is alive with nourishment and will dazzle you with mini-explosions of flavor.

2 **tablespoons (30 ml) expeller-pressed coconut oil**

1 **medium red onion, chopped**

2 **cloves garlic, finely chopped**

1 **inch (2.5 cm)-long piece fresh ginger, peeled and finely grated**

1 **small chile pepper, seeded and finely chopped**

8 **ounces (225 g) tempeh, cubed**

1 **cup (235 ml) chicken or vegetable stock**

1 **cup (100 g) chopped cauliflower**

1 **cup (71 g) chopped broccoli**

½ **pound (225 g) snap peas, fresh or frozen**

½ **cup (75 g) chopped cilantro**

½ **cup (8 g) chopped basil**

1 **cup (100 g) thinly sliced scallions**

2 **cups (475 ml) coconut milk**

1 **tablespoon (6.5 g) curry powder**

½ **teaspoon fish sauce or fine sea salt**

In a large skillet over medium heat, melt the coconut oil. Add the onion, garlic, ginger, and chile pepper, and cook for 4 to 5 minutes, or until they start to sweat. Move them to the sides of the skillet, then add the tempeh and stock. Cook until the tempeh is browned on all sides Add the cauliflower and broccoli and cook for 2 to 3 minutes. Add the peas, cilantro, basil, scallions, and coconut milk. Let simmer for 10 minutes, stirring occasionally. Stir in the curry powder and fish sauce or sea salt before serving.

Yield: 4 servings, or about 5 cups (1182 g)

Tempeh is an excellent source of isoflavones, which are known to reduce the risk of certain types of cancer, particularly prostate and breast cancers. A 4-ounce (112-g) serving of tempeh provides more than one-third of the average daily protein requirement at only 225 calories per serving, which means it's unlikely to cause weight gain!

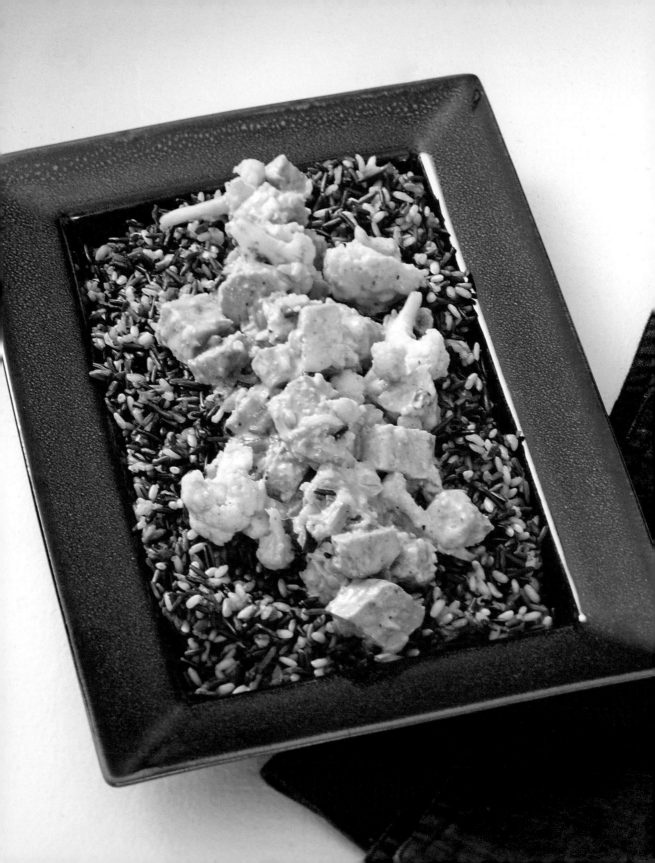

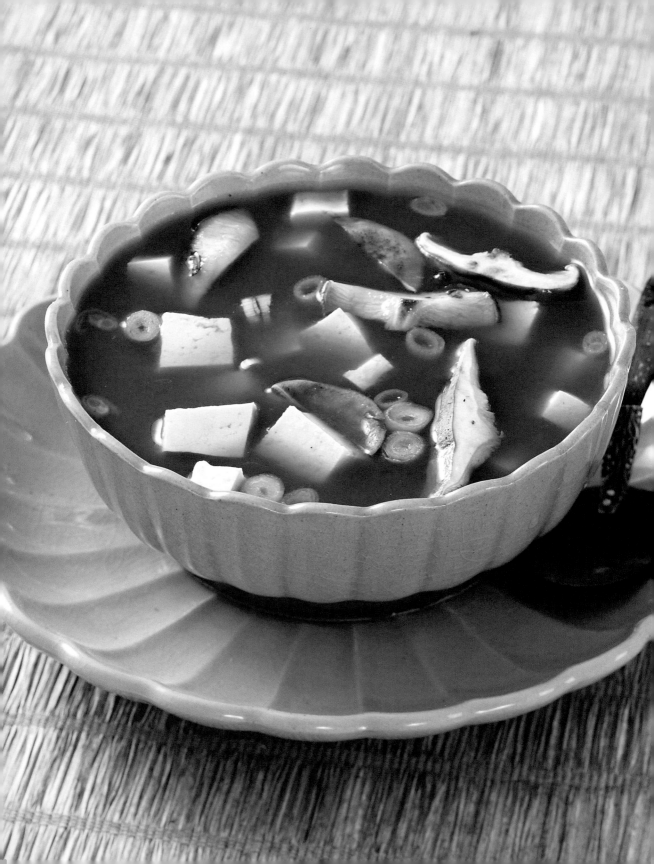

◀ Immune-Building Miso Soup with Tofu

Miso soup is a vital component of Japanese diets. Made from fermented soybeans, it's like chicken soup for the Japanese soul (but without the chicken). Through fermentation, the friendly flora break down soy's medicinal compounds—daidzein and genistein— which function as antioxidants and anti-inflammatory substances in the body. Miso also contains protein, fiber, tryptophan, manganese, vitamin K, and zinc. And it tastes delicious, too!

1 **tablespoon (1.3 g) dried seaweed (wakame works well)**

4 **cups (946 ml) dashi, chicken, vegetable, or fish stock**

¼ **cup (64 g) miso paste (any color)**

2 **tablespoons (12 g) thinly sliced scallions**

½ **cup (35 g) sliced shiitake or enoki mushrooms**

½ **cup (115 g) cubed, organic firm silken tofu**

In a small bowl, soak the seaweed in water for 10 minutes. Drain. In a medium saucepan over medium heat, bring the dashi or stock just to a simmer. Remove from the heat. Whisk in 2 tablespoons (32 g) of the miso paste until it is fully dissolved, then add the remaining 2 tablespoons (32 g) and dissolve. Dress with scallions, mushrooms, and tofu. Serve immediately.

Yield: 4 cups (946 ml)

For-the-Love-of-Sourdough Bread

What's not to love about the assertive, sour flavor and mild tang of fermented sourdough bread? The crust is soft and chewy, and the center is moist. Change the flavors by adding herbs, spices, fruits, or nuts of your choice. Serve it with fermented jams or relishes to increase probiotics and aid digestion.

1 **cup (235 ml) sourdough starter (see Resources)**

1 **cup (235 ml) warm filtered water**

1 **tablespoon (20 g) locally harvested raw honey (optional)**

1 **teaspoon fine sea salt**

3 **cups (330 g) sifted whole wheat or spelt flour**

½ **cup (30 g) finely chopped parsley (optional)**

In a bowl, combine the sourdough starter, water, honey, salt, flour, and parsley and blend into a smooth dough. Turn out onto a lightly floured board and knead for 3 minutes. Shape into an oval loaf with your hands and place onto a greased baking sheet. Cover and let rise for 1 to 2 hours, or until doubled in size.

Preheat the oven to 400°F (200°C, or gas mark 6). Spritz the dough with water, then, with a very sharp knife, cut an X into the loaf, about ¼ to ½ inch (6–13 mm) deep. Bake for 30 to 40 minutes, or until the crust is firm and golden, and the internal temperature of the loaf is about 200°F (93°C). (Insert the thermometer into the bottom or very low side of the loaf, so you don't mar your gorgeous creation!)

Yield: 1 loaf

Symbiotic Sourdough Pancakes

Easy to digest, these pancakes are so light they will melt in your mouth. The two organisms, wild yeast and bacteria, act in symbiosis to transform the wheat grain, making it more healthful and more digestible. These pancakes are ideal for people with wheat or "yeast" allergies and who usually have no problem eating sourdough. They taste sensational.

¾ **cup (180 ml) sourdough starter (see Resources)**

2½ **cups (313 g) whole wheat or gluten-free flour**

1 **cup (235 ml) sour milk or coconut kefir**

1 **teaspoon fine sea salt**

2 **eggs**

Spices of your choice (optional)

3 **tablespoons (45 ml) extra-virgin olive oil or coconut oil**

1 **teaspoon baking soda**

1 **large ripe banana, mashed**

In a large bowl, combine the sourdough starter, flour, and milk or kefir until thoroughly mixed. Allow the mixture to sit on the counter, covered with a clean towel, for 8 hours, or preferably overnight.

Punch down the dough, if it has risen, and mix in the salt, eggs, and any spices you wish to use until a batter is formed.

Heat the olive or coconut oil in a skillet or griddle over medium heat. Meanwhile, fold the baking soda gently into the batter, which will begin to gently foam and rise. Let it bubble and foam a minute or two, then add the mashed banana. Pour ⅓ cup (80 ml) batter into the hot oil. When bubbles appear at the center of the pancake (about 4 minutes), flip it over and cook the remaining side for about 2 minutes more. Remove from the heat and keep warm. Repeat until all the batter is used.

Serve with your favorite toppings. Yogurt, crème fraîche, maple syrup, or fermented jams (Probiotic Berry-Good-for-You Jam, (page 121) and butters (Fiber-Filled Fig and Apricot Honey Butter, page (124) work well.

Yield: Four to six 6-inch (15-cm) pancakes

Note This pancake recipe is a good way to use some of your extra sourdough starter. You may need to adjust this batter slightly by adding more liquid if it's too thick.

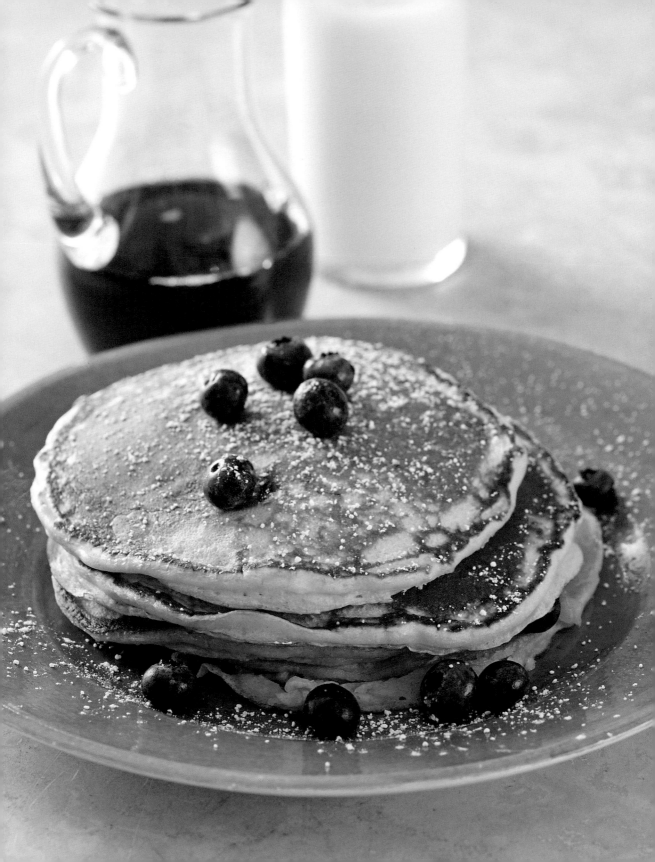

Easily Digestible Pizza Dough

Pizza is a Friday night favorite in my household and has been for years. I've adapted my favorite pizza dough recipe to include soaking the grains and adding whey, which makes it more easily digestible and nutritious because the minerals and vitamins are made more accessible to the body. Feel free to experiment by adding your own favorite herbs and spices into the mix. Then add toppings of cheese, chicken, tomatoes, or whatever you fancy. It is easy and delicious.

1 cup (235 ml) warm filtered water

1 tablespoon (20 g) locally harvested raw honey

1 tablespoon (15 ml) extra-virgin olive oil

3 tablespoons (45 ml) Easy Whey (page T92)

4 cups (500 g) whole wheat or spelt flour, plus extra for kneading

1 teaspoon fine sea salt

1 teaspoon dried basil

1 teaspoon dried oregano

1 teaspoon onion powder

1 tablespoon (12 g) instant yeast

On the night before you want to serve your pizza, combine the water, honey, olive oil, and whey in a large bowl. Blend in the 4 cups (500 g) flour. Cover with a clean towel and let sit on a counter for 12 to 24 hours.

The next day, add the salt, basil, oregano, onion powder, and yeast. Mix all the ingredients in the bowl with your hands until the dough pulls away from the sides. Transfer to a well-floured surface and knead for 10 minutes, adding flour as needed to keep it from sticking together.

Preheat the oven to 350°F (180°C, or gas mark 4). Gather the dough with your hands and press into a ball. Divide in half and role each piece into a 13-inch (33-cm) circle. Brush lightly with olive oil and place on a pizza pan. Turn up the edges ½ inch (13 mm) and pinch. Bake for 8 to 10 minutes, or until golden in color. Remove from the oven, add desired toppings, and bake for an additional 10 minutes.

Yield: Two 13-inch (33-cm) pizza crusts (or several smaller ones, as desired)

Soaking the grains breaks down phytic acid and complex carbohydrate molecules, which can cause intestinal gas. More B-complex vitamins are released through soaking or sprouting.

Strengthening Spinach Hummus

Rich in fiber and protein, chickpea hummus is loaded with vitamins and minerals such as calcium, zinc, and magnesium. Fermenting it with whey adds probiotics to make it super healthy.

2 **cups (400 g) dried garbanzo beans, or canned beans, rinsed and drained**

2 **tablespoons (30 ml) raw apple cider vinegar**

2 **tablespoons (30 ml) Easy Whey (page 92)**

1 **cup (60 g) fresh spinach, coarsely chopped**

3 **cloves fermented or regular garlic**

6 **tablespoons (90 ml) extra-virgin olive oil**

¼ **cup (60 ml) fresh lemon juice**

Dash of cayenne pepper

1 **teaspoon ground cumin (optional)**

2 **to 3 tablespoons (30–45 g) raw tahini**

½ **teaspoon fine sea salt**

In a medium bowl, soak the garbanzo beans in water and apple cider vinegar for 12 hours, or until sprouted. Drain. Place the sprouted beans, whey, spinach, garlic, olive oil, lemon juice, cayenne, and cumin in the bowl of a food processor and process until smooth. Add the tahini and salt and mix well. Refrigerate and serve cold.

Yield: 2½ cups (570 ml)

Spinach is loaded with vitamin A that not only protects and strengthens "entry points" into the human body, such as mucous membranes that line the respiratory and intestinal tracts, but is also a key component of lymphocytes (white blood cells) that fight infection.

Note Hummus serves as a great dip with raw veggies or as a delicious spread on wraps and sandwiches. It can also be easily turned into a tasty salad dressing by blending some hummus with water or stock until you get your desired drizzling consistency.

Dynamic Baked Beans

Beans (legumes) are often called "the poor people's meat"; however, they might be better known as the "healthy people's meat" because of their impressive health benefits. Baked beans have been a family favorite for many years. Sprouting and fermenting them makes them even more nutritious and improves their digestibility. Enjoy them for their buttery texture and nutty flavor, and know that you're getting a big boost of fiber, protein, minerals, and phytonutrients with every bite.

1 pound and 1½ ounces (496 g) dried white beans

3 (3 L) quarts filtered water, divided

4 to 5 tablespoons (60–75 ml) Easy Whey (page 92) or yogurt

1 onion, finely chopped

1 tablespoon (15 ml) raw apple cider vinegar

1 teaspoon fine sea salt

¼ cup (63 g) tomato purée

2 to 3 tablespoons (30–45 ml) maple syrup or molasses

Dash of cayenne pepper

Dash of black pepper

5 bay leaves

1 sprig rosemary

Dash of dried thyme

2 whole cloves

3½ ounces (98 g) unsalted butter

In a large bowl of nonchlorinated water, soak the beans for 12 to 24 hours, changing the soaking water after 12 hours. Rinse the beans well in cold water, then drain. Transfer the beans to a clean jar and cover with 1½ quarts (1420 ml) of the filtered water, then add the whey or yogurt and let them ferment in a cool spot at room temperature for 4 to 5 days; cover with a clean towel or cloth. Drain and rinse. The beans are ready to cook or can be refrigerated for later use (up to 2 to 3 days).

Preheat the oven to 300°F (150°C, or gas mark 2). Place the fermented beans in a 2-quart (2-L) bean pot or casserole dish and add the remaining 1½ quarts (1420 ml) filtered water and the onion, vinegar, salt, tomato purée, maple syrup or molasses, cayenne pepper, black pepper, bay leaves, rosemary, thyme, cloves, and butter. Cover and bake, stirring occasionally, for 3 to 4 hours, or until the beans are tender. If the water evaporates before the beans are ready, add more. If, at the end of cooking, there is too much water left, remove the lid and leave the pot in the oven 15 to 20 minutes at 325°F (170°C, or gas mark 3). Serve hot or cold. Baked beans will keep in the refrigerator for up to 2 months.

Yield: About 1½ quarts (1420 ml)

Note These baked beans go well with barbecued meats and fish and make a hearty side dish to almost anything.

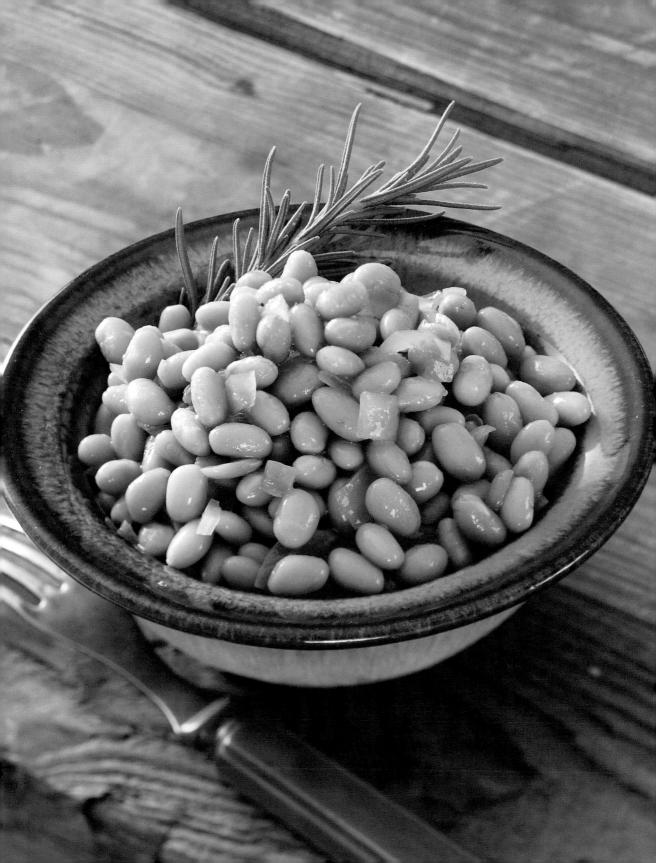

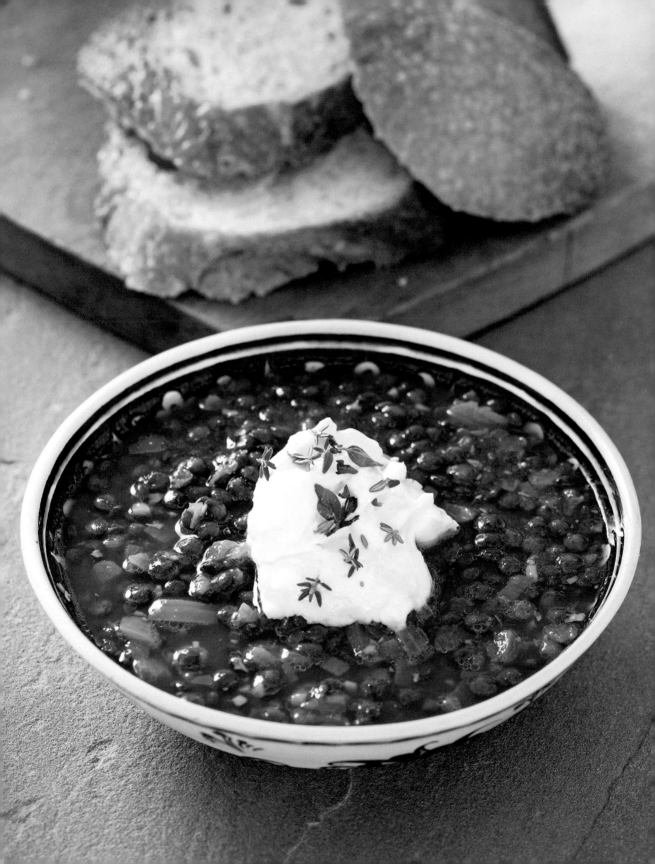

Love-Your-Heart Lentil Dal

This simple dal is one of my favorite go-to recipes because it is made with all pantry staples, is quick and easy to prepare, and has delicious flavors that are enhanced by fermentation.

1 cup (170 g) Lacto-Fermented Lentils (page 131)

3½ cups (830 ml) vegetable stock or filtered water, divided

1 tablespoon (15 ml) sesame oil or extra-virgin olive oil

1 cup (160 g) finely chopped onion

2 cloves garlic, finely chopped

1 tablespoon (6 g) finely chopped fresh ginger

3½ tablespoons (3.5 g) finely chopped cilantro, divided

1 teaspoon ground cumin

1 teaspoon ground turmeric

1 teaspoon fine sea salt

3 to 4 tablespoons (48–64 g) tomato paste

Dash of cayenne pepper

1 to 2 tablespoons (15–30 ml) fresh lemon juice, or to taste

In a medium saucepan over medium-high heat, bring the lentils and half the stock or water to a boil. Reduce the heat to low and simmer, covered, stirring occasionally, for about 20 to 30 minutes, or until the lentils are tender. Drain and set aside.

In a separate pot, heat the oil over medium-high heat. Add the onion, garlic, and ginger. Cook until the onion is translucent, about 5 minutes. Stirring constantly, add the remaining half of the water or stock, cooked lentils, ½ tablespoon (0.5 g) of the cilantro, cumin, turmeric, salt, tomato paste, and cayenne. Sauté until the lentils are well coated with the spices, about 3 minutes. Stir in the remaining 3 tablespoons (3 g) cilantro and the lemon juice. Cook several minutes more until the dal is of a desired consistency, adding more stock or water if needed. Taste, and the adjust seasonings. Serve hot with sourdough bread (see page 135) and garnish with a dollop of yogurt, if desired.

Yield: About 3½ cups (563 g)

Want to keep your heart happy? Eat lentils. They're well known for their cholesterol-lowering fiber, but that's not the only nutritional benefit that these little wonders supply. Lentils contain significant amounts of folate and magnesium, both of which support heart health.

Note Uncooked lentils have a shelf life. Store them in an airtight container in a cool, dry, and dark place for up to 12 months.

Wholesome Tempeh Burgers

Enjoy the super-nutritious benefits of this amazingly delicious tempeh burger,
which delivers a wild nutty flavor with a firm yet tender, meaty texture.

1 **package (8 ounces, or 225 g) organic tempeh, cut into cubes**

¼ **onion, finely chopped**

½ **cup (120 g) grated zucchini**

1 **tablespoon (15 ml) extra-virgin olive oil, plus additional for frying**

1 **tablespoon (2.5 g) minced fresh basil, or 1 teaspoon dried**

1 **tablespoon (3 g) dried oregano**

2 **tablespoons (8 g) finely chopped fresh parsley**

½ **teaspoon fine sea salt**

8 **slices For-the-Love-of-Sourdough Bread (page 135)**

4 **tablespoons (60 ml) mayonnaise (preferably fermented)**

1 **cup (142 g) sauerkraut**

4 **slices Swiss cheese**

4 **leaves romaine lettuce**

1 **cup (50 g) alfalfa sprouts**

Place the tempeh in the bowl of a food processor and process until finely chopped. Transfer to a large mixing bowl, and add the onion, zucchini, olive oil, basil, oregano, parsley, and salt. Blend with a fork until it is evenly mixed. Divide the mixture into 4 portions and roll into balls, then flatten into patties.

To prepare the burgers, fry in a lightly oiled skillet over medium heat until browned on both sides and firm to the touch. Or, if desired, bake in a 350°F (180°C, or gas mark 4) oven for about 20 minutes, flipping halfway through. Remove when lightly browned and firm to the touch.

To serve, lay each patty on a slice of sourdough bread spread with 1 tablespoon (15 ml) mayonnaise. Top with ¼ cup (35 g) sauerkraut, 1 slice Swiss cheese, 1 romaine leaf, ¼ cup (13 g) alfalfa sprouts, and a second slice of bread.

Yield: 4 burgers

Note The starter culture in tempeh is Rhizopus oligosporus, *a friendly filamentous fungi. As the culture spores germinate, they bind the soybeans together into compact white cakes.*

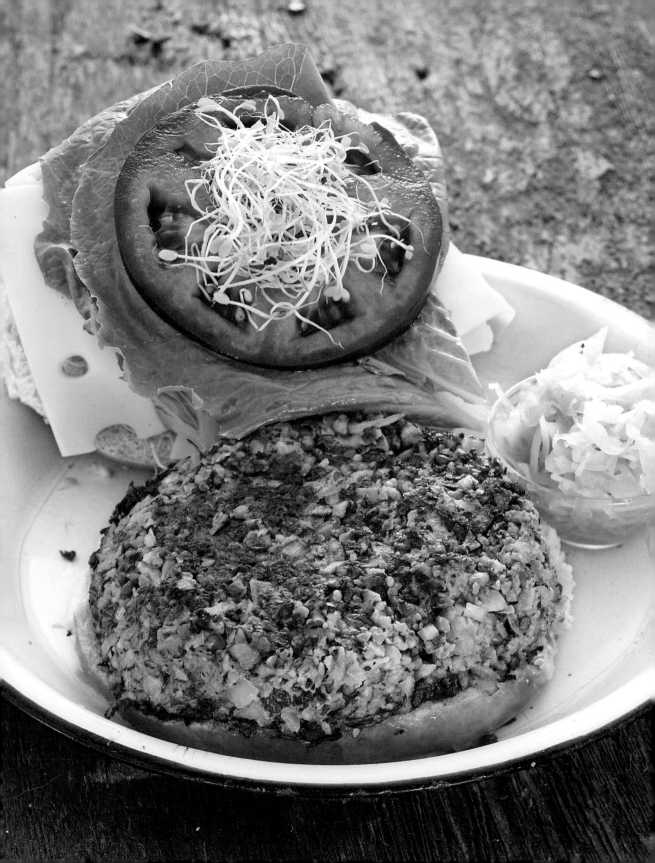

Protein-Powered Pinto Beans

If you're wondering how to replace red meat in your menus, then become a fan of pinto beans. These hearty beans are a good source of protein, which is made complete when you combine the beans with whole grains, like rice. Fermenting them adds precious probiotics for improved digestion. Pinto beans also contain a generous amount of fiber to support prebiotics.

2   **cups (400 g) dried pinto beans**

1   **large onion, chopped**

3   **cloves garlic, minced**

1   **teaspoon fine sea salt**

¼   **cup (60 ml) Easy Whey (page 92)**

½   **to 1 cup (120–235 ml) Basic Brine (page 92)**

Place the beans in a large bowl of nonchlorinated water, and soak for 12 to 24 hours, changing the water after 12 hours. Rinse the beans well in cold water, then drain. Add the beans to a medium saucepan, cover with water, and cook over medium-low heat until tender. Drain and let cool.

In a large bowl, add the pinto beans, onion, garlic, salt, and whey, and stir until well mixed. Pour the mixture into a 1-quart (946-ml) fermenting jar. Add enough of the brine to completely cover the beans, leaving 1 inch (2.5 cm) of space from the top, then cap the jar tightly. Leave the jar in a dark spot in your kitchen at room temperature for 3 days. Refrigerate and use within 60 days. You can serve these beans with salad greensor steamed vegetables, or add to your stir-fries.

Yield: 4½ cups (770 g)

Energy-Boosting Granola Bars

1   **cup (160 g) steel-cut oats or (80 g) rolled oats**

1   **cup (178 g) dates, pitted and chopped**

1   **cup (235 ml) Easy Whey (page 92) or kefir (or coconut kefir)**

½   **cup (80 g) brown rice flour, plus more for dusting pan**

½   **cup (40 g) unsweetened shredded coconut**

½   **cup (73 g) almonds, chopped**

3   **tablespoons (24 g) sesame seeds**

½   **tablespoon fine sea salt**

1   **tablespoon (7 g) ground cinnamon**

1   **cup (260 g) sugar-free peanut butter**

½   **cup (170 g) maple syrup**

Grind the oats in a blender or food processor until they are ground into a coarse flour. In a large bowl, mix together the oat flour, dates, whey or kefir, brown rice flour, coconut, almonds, and sesame seeds. Add the salt and cinnamon and mix well. Cover with a clean towel and let set for 6 to 8 hours.

Preheat the oven to 75°F (24°C). (You can set it as high as 100°F [38°C], but if your oven doesn't go this low, use a food dehydrator, which allows you to set the temperature lower.) Add the peanut butter and maple syrup to the oat mixture and stir well. Dust a 9 x 13-inch (23 x 33-cm) pan with flour, and spread the mixture over the entire surface, pressing into the corners. Bake the granola for 8 to 10 hours, or until the granola bars are the consistency you like, whether crunchy or gooey. Cut the bars into squares and eat immediately or refrigerate. The bars will keeps for several months.

Yield: 12 to 16 bars

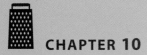

CHAPTER 10

(Non-) Dairy, Meat, and Fish

Many of the recipes in this chapter use kefir. Kefir is a milk product made from a culture starter community of kefir grains added to the fermenting liquid. The culture community can be added to cow, goat, or coconut milk. Kefir is considered superior to yogurt because it offers a greater number of beneficial strains of bacteria and is more easily digested.

There are two types of kefir grains: water and milk. They are not actual grains, per se, but merely resemble them. Both types of grains are similar in that they both consist of lactic acid bacteria and yeast existing in a symbiotic relationship, and they provide all of the same health benefits. The main difference is that water kefir grains allow you to make probiotic foods without dairy; they can be used with sugar water, fruit juice, and coconut water. This is beneficial to those who are vegan or prefer a completely dairy-free diet. You can use milk kefir grains with cow or goat milk, soy milk, or coconut milk. Both grains can be stored and used repeatedly. Store your milk kefir grains in a glass jar in a small amount of milk (preferably organic). Use about twice to several times the amount of liquid as grains. Store water kefir grains in a glass jar in a small amount of water, about twice to several times the amount of liquid as grains, but add 1 or 2 tablespoons (15 or 30 ml) of sugar to feed the grains. Store at room temperature or in the refrigerator, changing the liquid every few days if kept at room temperature and weekly if refrigerated.

Bone-Building Fermented Sour Cream

Smooth, creamy, divinely delicious, and highly nutritious, fresh sour cream made from the cream of grass-fed cows is one of life's greatest pleasures. It's loaded with calcium made more available to your body by the fermentation process. Add it to tacos, soups, nachos, and just about anything else you wish.

1 or 2 tablespoons (30 ml) organic sour cream

2 tablespoons (30 ml) Easy Whey starter culture (See Resources, page 204)

2 cups (460 ml) cream (preferably raw cream from grass-fed cows)

Stir together the sour cream and starter culture. Add the sour cream mixture and cream to a 1-quart (946-ml) fermenting jar and mix well. Cover the jar with a cloth and secure with a rubber band. Leave at room temperature for 12 to 24 hours, until it sets like firm yogurt. Cover with a lid and refrigerate for at least 6 hours before using. Store the refrigerator, where it will keep for several weeks.

Yield: 2 cups (460 ml)

Note Eat ¼ cup (60 g) of this sour cream, and you will take in 26 percent of the phosphorus your body requires each day for bone health.

Easy Kefir Cheese ▶

Easy to make, loaded with B vitamins, and rich in probiotics, this silky-soft kefir cheese is great as a dip with vegetables or spread over sourdough bread or crackers.

1 quart (946 ml) plain kefir

½ teaspoon fine sea salt

Line a colander with cheesecloth and set it inside a bowl. Pour the kefir into the cheesecloth and tie up the ends. Let sit for 12 to 24 hours, depending on the consistency desired. The longer you leave it, the more whey drips into the bowl and the thicker and more sour the cheese becomes. Untie the cheesecloth and scrape the cheese into a storage container. Mix in the salt. Transfer the cheese to the refrigerator, where it will keep for several weeks.

Yield: 2 cups (460 g)

Note Change the consistency from creamy cheese to a harder cheese by draining for more than 12 hours. The longer you leave it, the firmer it becomes. Add nuts, herbs, and spices when you add the salt, to flavor your cheese.

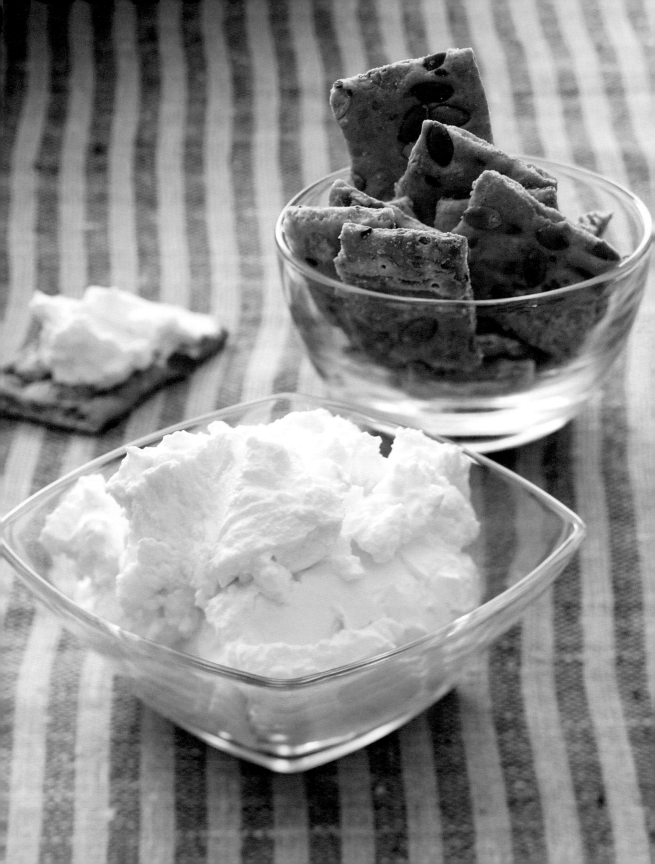

Probiotic-Rich Kefir Cream

Enjoy the tart, refreshing flavor and the slight effervescent, zesty tang of this healthful delight. Kefir is naturally made up of more than a dozen Lactobacilli bacteria *species and various yeasts, offering you the benefits of multiple live probiotics that happily coexist. And kefir is much more digestible than yogurt is.*

2 cups (460 ml) heavy cream (preferably raw cream from grass-fed cows)

1 tablespoon (30 g) milk kefir grains (see Resources)

Pour the cream into a wide-mouth 1-pint (473-ml) jar and gently stir in the kefir grains. Allow them to float freely. Cover the jar with cloth and secure with a rubber band. Let it sit at room temperature for 12 to 24 hours, until it sets like firm yogurt. Scoop out the grains, and if not reusing them right away, place them in fresh milk or water in the refrigerator to keep them alive for later use. Cover with a lid and refrigerate for 6 to 8 hours before using. It will keep in the refrigerator for several weeks.

Yield: 2 cups (475 ml)

Note You can add a dollop of this nutritious cream to smoothies or soups, or spoon over baked or mashed potatoes.

Blood-Sugar-Balancing Coconut Milk Kefir ▶

This recipe turns coconut milk into a healthful, probiotic-rich beverage. It makes a delicious alternative to cow or goat milk kefir.

1 tablespoon (30 g) milk or water kefir grains (see Resources)

1½ cups (355 ml) coconut milk

Add the milk kefir grains to the coconut milk, and allow the milk to culture for 12 to 48 hours, until the desired consistency and taste is achieved. Remove the kefir grains and place them in fresh milk or water in the refrigerator to keep them alive for later use.

Yield: 1½ cups (355 ml)

The essential fatty acids in coconut milk help keep blood sugar levels balanced. Coconut milk is also rich in phosphorus, which is an essential nutrient the body needs to strengthen bones.

Note Coconut kefir has a variety of uses: as a base for ice cream or smoothies, as an addition to coffee, as "milk" poured over granola, and as a dairy replacement in recipes such as sauces and delicious curries.

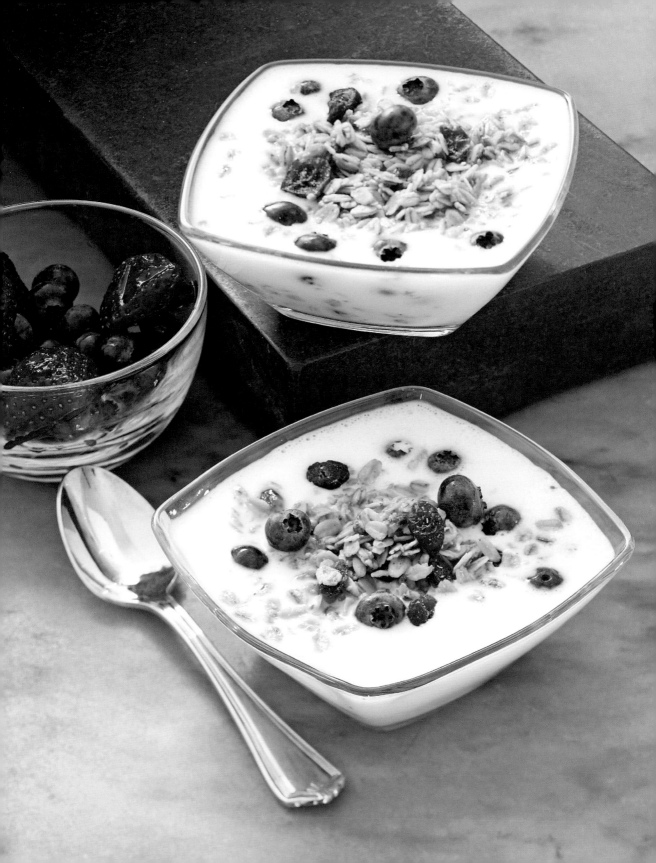

Russian Cucumber-Kefir Soup

This recipe came from provincial Russia around the turn of the twentieth century. It was served to the czars of Russia in their palace and was considered a delicacy. The peasants got the recipe from relatives who served in the palace. It is being passed on to you with a big difference: originally made with buttermilk, it's here been updated to include kefir. Many thanks to a dear friend, Faithful To Jesus (her real name), who passed it on to me! Served ice cold—even with ice cubes in the bowl—on a hot summer afternoon, little else can refresh so well.

1 **large (or 2 medium) seedless cucumbers, grated, with peels left on**

1 **large (or 2 medium) tomatoes, finely chopped**

1 **medium (or 2 small) skin-on boiled potatoes, chopped**

½ **cup (30 g) finely chopped parsley**

2 **large hard-boiled eggs, finely chopped**

¼ **cup (38 g) finely chopped red, yellow, or green bell pepper**

5 **to 7 scallions, finely chopped**

2 **to 3 teaspoons (2.6–3.9 g) finely chopped fresh dill, or 1 to 2 teaspoons dried**

1 **to 3 cups (235–705 ml) kefir**

In a large bowl, combine the cucumber, tomato, potato, parsley, eggs, bell pepper, scallions, and dill. Cover with a lid and refrigerate for 24 hours for the flavors to meld.

About an hour before you are ready to serve, add 1 cup (235 ml) kefir and stir. Judge its thickness and flavor, and add more kefir to your liking. Refrigerate until ready to serve.

Serve ice cold. Allow people to season their individual servings with salt and pepper. If seasoned in advance, the salt will draw water out of the cucumber, causing the soup to become thinner.

Yield: About 1 quart (946 ml)

Note This is such a forgiving recipe. If you don't have an ingredient listed, just leave it out or add something else you like; just adjust the quantities to what looks or tastes right to you.

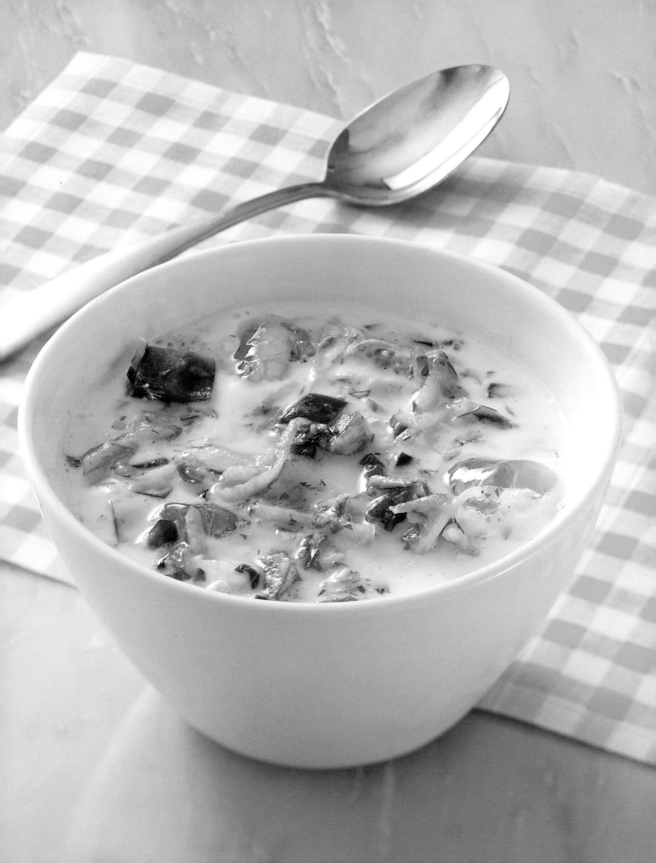

Cooling Carrot and Celery Kefir

With this cooling, power-food combination, you get vitamin A and a host of other important health benefits, including cancer prevention, beautiful skin, and antiaging effects, as well as celery's anti-inflammatory properties.

¼ **cup (60 ml) fresh carrot juice**

¼ **cup (60 ml) fresh celery juice**

¾ **cup (175 ml) plain kefir**

Dash of cayenne pepper (optional)

Put the carrot juice, celery juice, kefir, and cayenne into the container of a blender and blend until smooth.

Yield: 1 serving, or 1¼ cups (285 ml)

Note During dry or hot weather, drink a glass of this elixir between meals. It helps normalize body temperature, replenish electrolytes, and promote healthy kidney function, and it's loaded with probiotics to strengthen immune responses.

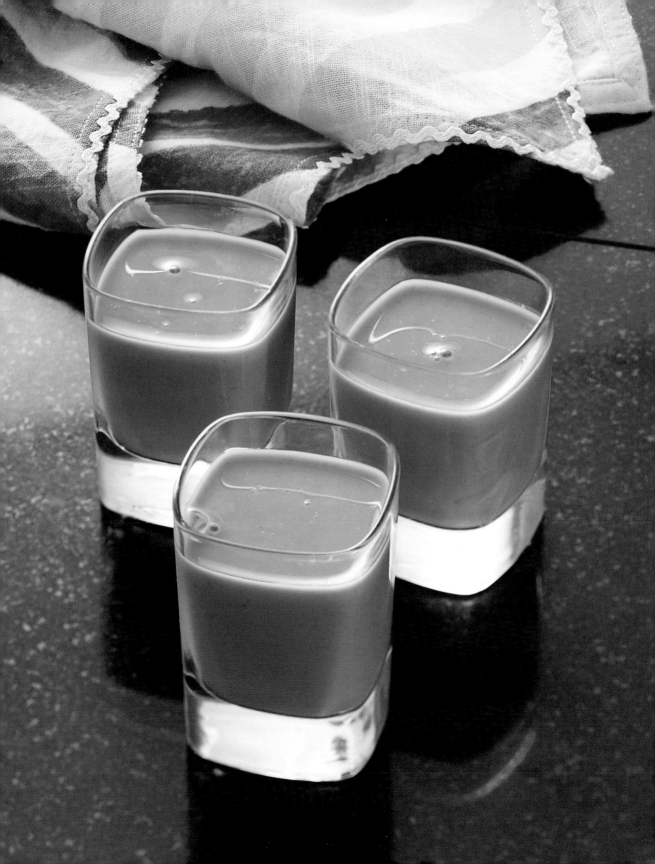

Glowing Papaya Kefir Ice Cream

Papaya is full of fiber and enzymes for healthy digestion and is very high in antioxidants and essential minerals. Blended with kefir, it makes a deliciously rich combination for an unforgettable ice cream that's beneficial in every way.

1 **cup (175 g) chopped papaya**

2 **eggs**

¾ **cup (150 g) unrefined sugar, or ¼ cup (85 g) locally harvested raw honey**

2 **cups (475 ml) plain kefir, yogurt, buttermilk, or whole milk**

1 **cup (235 ml) Probiotic-Rich Kefir Cream (page 150) or non-kefir heavy cream**

2 **teaspoons vanilla extract**

Place the papaya, eggs, and sugar in the container of a blender and blend. Add the kefir, kefir cream, and vanilla, and blend. Transfer to an ice cream maker and follow the instructions that go with the machine.

Yield: About 1 quart (946 ml)

Papaya is used in many face packs and skin-lightening creams because it contains the enzyme papain, which helps dissolve dead skin, thus imparting a fresh and clean glow to the face.

Note Add different fruits or coconut to flavor according to your taste.

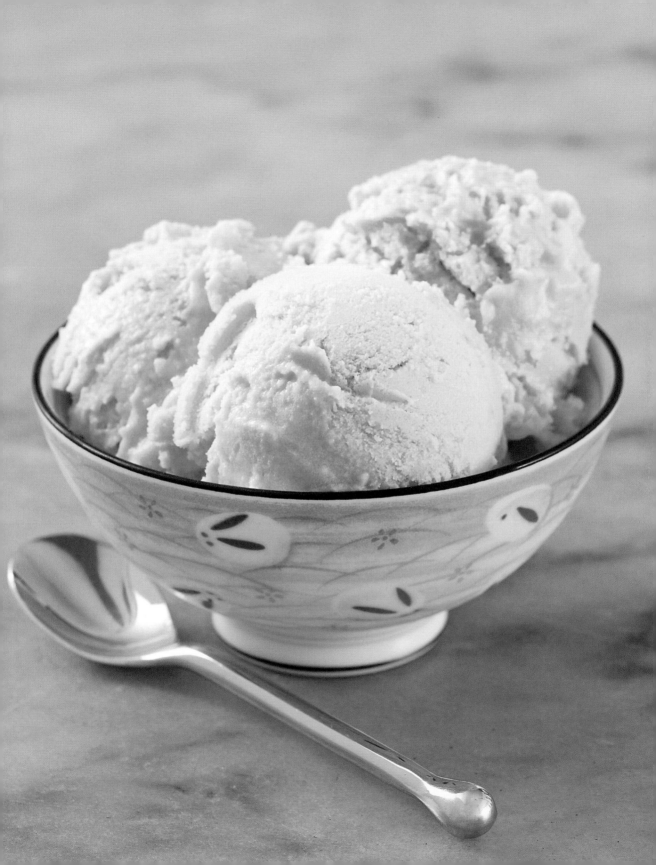

Refreshing Orange Coconut Kefir Smoothie

Abundant in vitamins, minerals, enzymes, and probiotics, this morning citrus drink is a great replacement for orange juice. You'll soon be looking forward to your daily health drink that's loaded with probiotics.

1 **cup (235 ml) plain fresh kefir**

1 **orange, peeled and seeded**

1 **egg yolk (preferably organic)**

¼ **cup (20 g) shredded coconut**

1 **tablespoon (20 g) locally harvested raw honey, or 1 date, pitted**

1 **teaspoon vanilla extract**

1 **or 2 ice cubes**

Place the kefir, orange, egg yolk, coconut, honey, vanilla extract, and ice cubes in the container of a blender and blend until smooth. Serve cold or at room temperature.

Yield: 1 serving, or 2 cups (475 ml)

Note Add different fruits or chocolate to change flavors.

Chocolate Cherry Kefir Smoothie ▶

Nothing complements the wonderful sharpness of cherries more than chocolate. This smoothie is topped off with the tangy, sour flavor of kefir and is loaded with probiotic goodness.

1 **cup (235 ml) plain kefir**

1 **small to medium ripe banana**

½ **cup (78 g) fresh or frozen cherries, pitted**

1 **tablespoon (7 g) cocoa powder or carob powder**

1 **or 2 ice cubes**

Dash of cayenne pepper (optional)

Place the kefir, banana, cherries, chocolate or carob, ice cubes, and cayenne in the container of a blender and blend until smooth. Serve cold or at room temperature.

Yield: 1 serving, or 1½ cups (355 ml)

Cherries are known as a "superfruit" because of their high content of antioxidants called anthocyanins, which support heart health and reduce the risk of cancer. They are also rich in vitamins C, E, and folate; the minerals potassium, magnesium, and iron; and fiber.

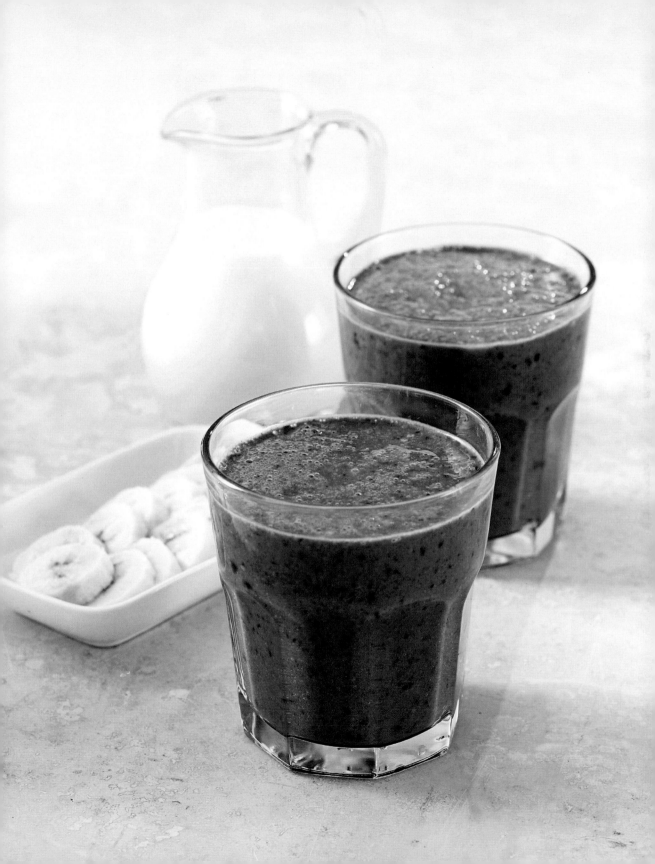

Stomach-Soothing Tzatziki Herb Sauce

Delightfully soothing on the stomach, tzatziki sauce gets its name from the Greeks, who spread it over souvlaki and on pita bread, and serve it over salads. The herbs and lemon give it a delicious tang, plus it's loaded with probiotic goodness.

1 cup (230 g) yogurt

1 cucumber, peeled and roughly chopped

2 tablespoons (30 ml) extra-virgin olive oil

Zest and juice of ½ an organic lemon

2 garlic cloves

2 tablespoons (12 g) chopped fresh mint

1 tablespoon (8 g) chopped fresh dill, or ½ tablespoon dried

½ teaspoon fine sea salt

Dash of cayenne pepper

Line a colander with cheesecloth and place it in a bowl. Pour the yogurt into the cheesecloth and tie up the ends. Let it drip for 2 to 4 hours, then scrape out the thickened yogurt. Retain the whey for future use.

Place the yogurt, cucumber, olive oil, lemon zest and juice, garlic, mint, dill, salt, and cayenne into the bowl of a food processor and mix well. Transfer to a serving dish, cover, and chill for several hours before serving so that the flavors meld together.

Yield: 1½ cups (355 ml)

Because of its active compounds, mint has been shown to relieve symptoms of indigestion and irritable bowel syndrome.

Note Zest the lemon first, then juice it.

Yogurt Kefir Ranch Dip

Nothing beats homemade ranch dressing, especially when it contains the creamy, tangy taste of kefir and yogurt. This dip is easy and quick to make.

¾ **cup (175 ml) kefir**

½ **cup (115 g) mayonnaise (preferably lacto-fermented mayonnaise, see page 176)**

2 **tablespoons (28 g) plain yogurt**

1 **teaspoon chopped dill**

2 **teaspoons chopped parsley**

1 **clove garlic, finely minced**

½ **teaspoon onion salt**

¼ **teaspoon freshly ground black pepper**

Line a colander with cheesecloth and set it inside a bowl. Pour the kefir into the cheesecloth and tie up the ends. Let it drip for 12 to 24 hours, or until it reaches the consistency of sour cream or slightly thicker. Untie the cheesecloth and scrape out the cheese. The ¾ cup (175 ml) kefir produces ½ cup (115 g) cheese.

In a small bowl, mix together the kefir, mayonnaise, and yogurt. Whisk in the dill, parsley, garlic, salt, and pepper, and transfer to a glass jar. Cover and refrigerate for at least 2 hours prior to serving so the flavors blend.

Yield: About 1¼ cups (285 ml)

Note *Enjoy this dip with veggie sticks, top it over salad greens, or add it to a sourdough sandwich. To enhance the flavor and nutrients, add half an avocado.*

Wild Mixed Berries Frozen Yogurt

Enjoy the rich, creamy, tart flavor of frozen yogurt, knowing that it's loaded with beneficial bacteria and antioxidants.

2 cups (290 g) fresh or frozen mixed berries (blackberry, strawberry, raspberry, or blueberry)

3 tablespoons (45 ml) milk

⅔ cup (230 g) locally harvested raw honey

2 cups (460 g) plain yogurt

1½ tablespoons (22 ml) vanilla extract

If using frozen berries, thaw first, retaining the juices. Mash the berries with a fork or purée in a blender. In a medium bowl, stir to combine the milk and honey. Add the berries to the milk and mix together. Add the yogurt and vanilla and combine. Transfer to an ice cream maker and follow the instructions that go with the machine.

Yield: About 1 quart (946 ml)

Note Homemade frozen yogurt is much healthier than store-bought because you can control the type and amount of sweetener. Many store-bought brands contain significant amounts of sugar, making them higher in calories as well as inflammatory.

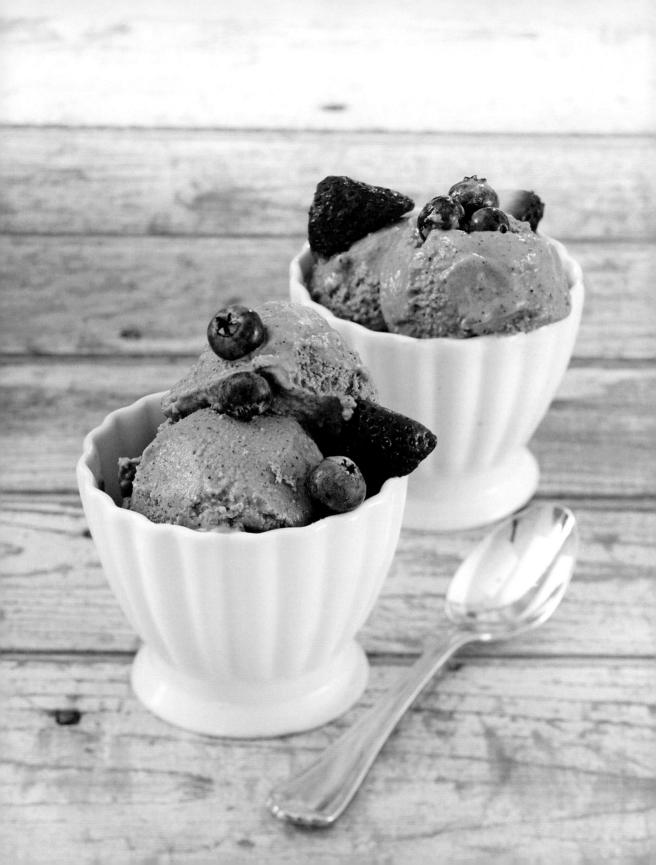

Brain-Protective Honey-Ginger Salmon

The omega-3s in salmon are greatly enhanced by fermentation. I've adapted this delicious recipe from Sally Fallon's book Nourishing Traditions. *For an added nutritional punch, serve it on sourdough bread with kefir cheese (see pages 135 and 148), or keep it simple and serve with a salad.*

1 **tablespoon (20 g) locally harvested raw honey**

1 **teaspoon chopped fresh ginger**

2 **or 3 scallions, chopped**

1 **teaspoon whole peppercorns**

¼ **cup (60 ml) Easy Whey (page 92)**

¼ **cup (60 ml) Basic Brine (page 92)**

1 **pound (455 g) salmon fillet, skinned and cut into bite-size pieces**

2 **slices lemon**

2 **tablespoons (8 g) chopped fresh dill**

2 **bay leaves**

In a medium bowl, combine the honey, ginger, scallions, peppercorns, whey, and brine. Pack the fish, lemon, and dill into a 1-quart (946-ml) fermenting jar. Pour the honey mixture over the fish so that the fish is completely submerged. Leave 1 inch (2.5 cm) of space below the top of the jar. Add the bay leaves and cap the jar tightly. Leave at room temperature for 24 hours. Transfer to the refrigerator, where it will keep for up to 2 weeks. Remove the salmon from the brine before serving

You can add this, as is, to salads, or serve it with vegetables. You can even add fermented relishes and other condiments to enhance probiotics and flavor

Yield: 1 pound (455 g)

Note Wild-caught (also called Pacific) salmon contains higher levels of omega-3 essential fatty acids and lower levels of bacteria than farmed salmon. PCBs and dioxins, which are endocrine disrupters, are also found in farmed salmon. Note that all Atlantic salmon is farmed.

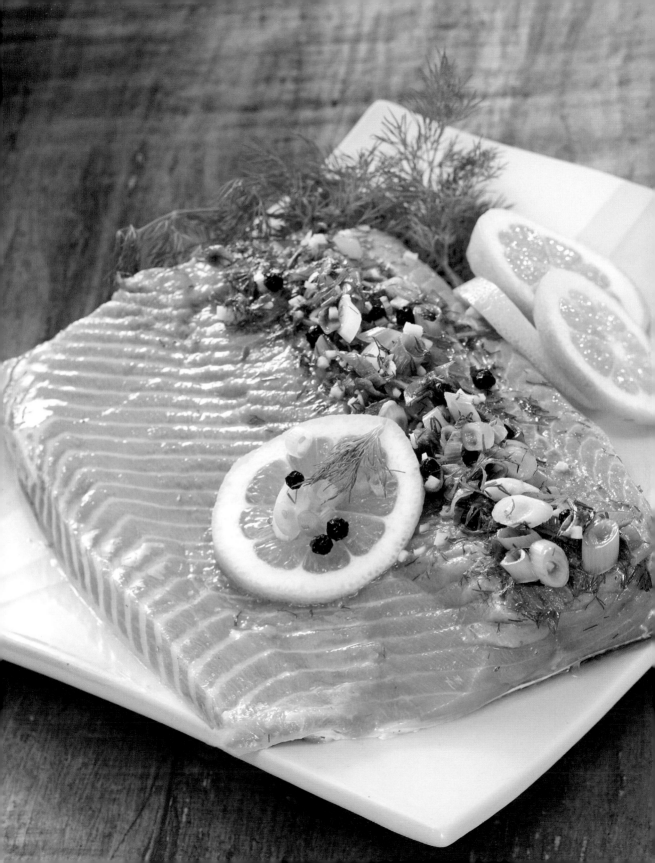

Strengthening Herbed Corned Beef

Moist and tender, corned beef is a good source of iron, which helps build red blood cells that carry oxygen throughout your body. It's also loaded with antioxidant vitamins A and C, which strengthen your immune system.

- 1 **tablespoon (20 g) unrefined sweetener (rapadura, raw honey, maple syrup)**
- 2 **tablespoons (12 g) freshly ground black pepper**
- 2 **tablespoons (10 g) freshly ground coriander seeds**
- 4½ **cups (1064 ml) Basic Brine (page 92)**
- 3 to 4 **(1.4–1.8 kg) grass-fed beef brisket, rump, or round, rinsed and cut into 2- to 3-inch (5–7.5-cm) chunks**
- 1 **small onion, quartered**
- 4 to 6 **cloves garlic**
- 2 **bay leaves**
- 1 **tablespoon (2.4 g) thyme**
- 1 **teaspoon fine sea salt**

In a medium saucepan over medium-low heat, combine the sweetener, pepper, coriander, and brine and heat gently until dissolved. Let cool to room temperature.

Pack the meat into one large or two small airlock fermenting containers. Pour the brine mixture over the meat and leave 1 inch (2.5 cm) of space at the top. Place a clean, flat, disk shaped object on top of the meat to hold it down under the brine weighted down with a clean rock or resealable plastic bag filled with water. Close the jar with an airlock. Leave in a dark spot in your kitchen at room temperature for 8 hours. Transfer to the refrigerator for 7 to 10 days. Check it daily and add more brine, as needed, to cover the meat.

When ready to cook it, drain the corned beef, and rinse well under cold running water. Place the beef in a large stockpot. Add the onion, garlic, bay leaves, thyme, and salt, and cover with water. Bring to a boil, then reduce the heat and simmer for 1½ to 2 hours, or until tender. Remove the beef and transfer to a serving dish. Discard the liquid when cool. The cooked beef will keep for up to 5 days stored in the refrigerator.

Yield: 3 to 4 pounds (1.4–1.8kg)

Note As an alternative to cooking on the stove, the corned beef can be cooked in the oven at 325°F (170°C, or gas mark 3) for 1 hour or in a slow cooker at medium setting (simmering heat) for approximately 1 hour. Either way, enjoy it piled high on rye or sourdough bread and topped with fermented mustard and sauerkraut to make a Reuben sandwich.

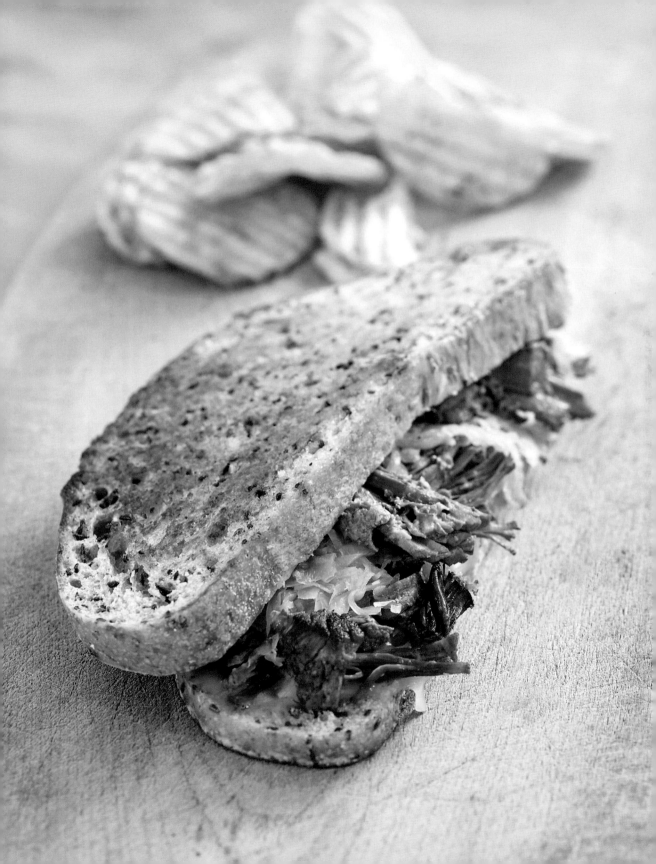

Fermented Mediterranean Mackerel

Rich with omega-3 essential fatty acids, selenium, and vitamin B12, mackerel is found in North Atlantic and Mediterranean waters. It's well known for its blood-thinning and heart-protective qualities. Its firm flesh lends itself nicely to fermentation.

1 **cup (235 ml) Basic Brine (page 92)**

¼ **cup (60 ml) Easy Whey (page 92)**

1 **to 2 tablespoons (5–10 g) whole black peppercorns**

1 **tablespoon (20 g) locally harvested raw honey**

1 **pound (455 g) mackerel fillet, skinned and cut into bite-size pieces**

2 **tablespoons (8 g) chopped fresh parsley**

2 **bay leaves**

1 **medium orange, sliced**

In a small bowl, combine the brine, whey, peppercorns, and honey. Pack the fish, parsley, and bay leaves into a 1-quart (946-ml) fermenting jar. Pour the brine mixture over the fish, making sure the fish is completely submerged. Add more brine, if necessary, to cover. Be sure the level of the liquid stays 1 inch (2.5 cm) below the jar rim. Add the orange slices. Cap the jar tightly and keep it at room temperature for 24 hours. Transfer it to the refrigerator, where it will keep for up to 2 weeks. Remove the mackerel from the brine before serving.

Yield: 1 pound (455 g)

Note When purchasing mackerel, look for those with shiny bodies and bright eyes. They should feel firm and rigid. Eat this dish with crackers, on sourdough, or alongside steamed or fermented vegetables.

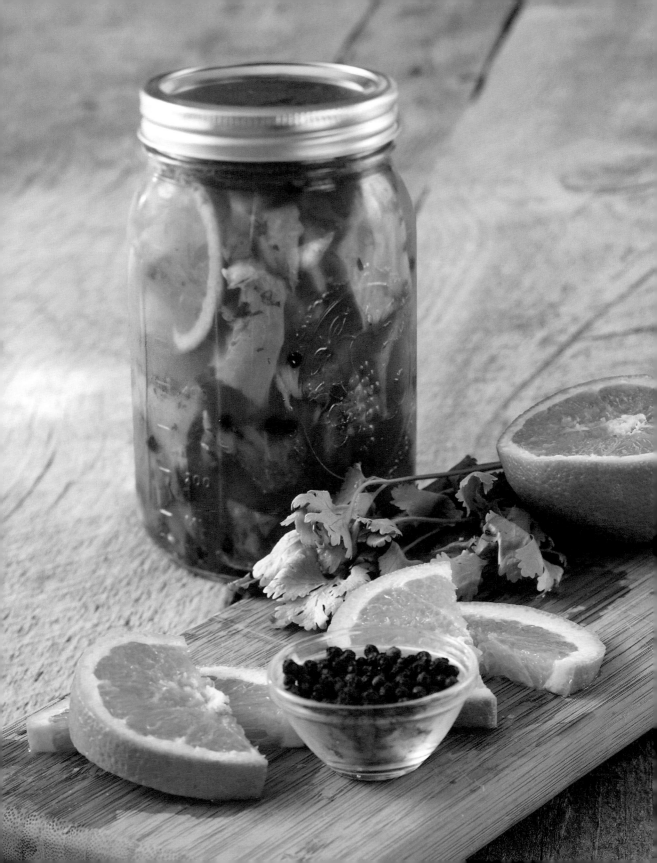

Artery-Protective Pickled Herring

This beloved, tasty delicacy is enjoyed in many parts of Europe and even into the Far East. Enjoy it with sliced red onions, brine-pickled carrots, rye sourdough toasts, hard-boiled eggs, freshly chopped dill, and a little horseradish cream sauce. It's simply delicious.

1 **cup (235 ml) Basic Brine (page 92)**

¼ **cup (60 ml) Easy Whey (page 92)**

⅓ **cup (80 ml) freshly squeezed lemon juice**

1 **tablespoon (11 g) mustard seeds, or 2 tablespoons (30 ml) prepared mustard**

1 **pound (455 g) skinless herring, cut into ½-inch (13-mm) pieces**

1 **small onion, coarsely chopped**

1 **or 2 large sprigs fresh dill, chopped**

1 **teaspoon allspice berries**

1 **teaspoon coriander seeds**

½ **teaspoon black pepper**

1 **bay leaf**

⅛ **teaspoon red pepper flakes**

In a small bowl, combine the brine, whey, lemon juice, and mustard. Place the herring, onion, dill, allspice, coriander, black pepper, bay leaf, and red pepper flakes in a wide-mouth 1-quart (946-ml) jar. Pour the brine mixture over all. Add more brine, if necessary, to cover, making sure the level of the liquid stays 1 inch (2.5 cm) below the jar rim. Cover the jar with a lid or an airlock, and leave at room temperature for 1 day. Transfer to the refrigerator, where it will keep for up to 2 weeks. Remove the herring from the brine before serving.

Yield: 1 pound (455 g)

Note Both herring and sardines are rich sources of EPA and DHA, which are omega-3 essential fatty acids renowned for their triglyceride-lowering, platelet-unsticking, and artery-protective effects.

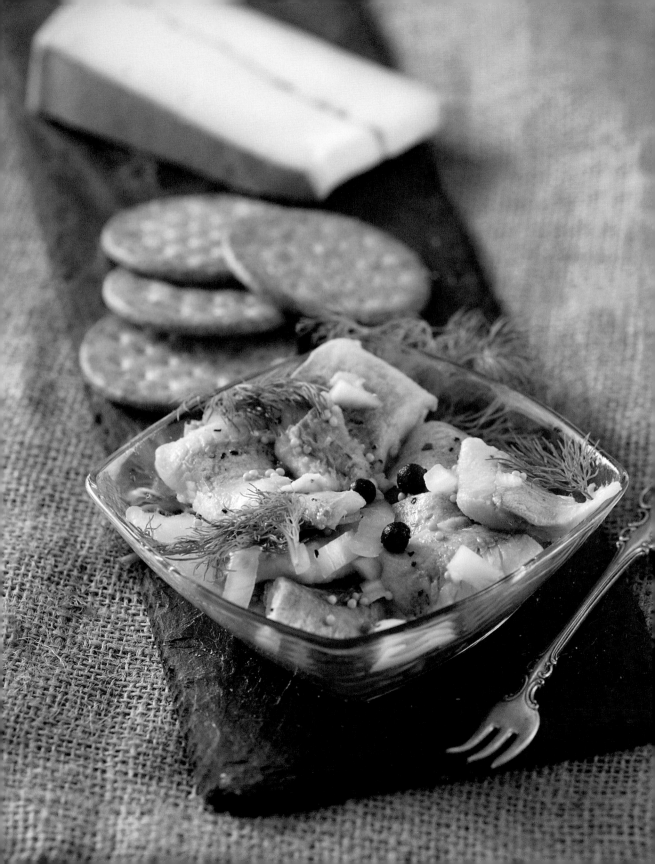

Bone-Building Fermented Fish Sauce

Fish sauce originated in Southeast Asia, where it is used in everyday cooking. It's high in calcium and rich in iodine to benefit the thyroid gland.

2 **cups (475 ml) filtered water**

3 **tablespoons (54 g) fine sea salt**

2 **bay leaves**

1 **teaspoon whole peppercorns**

1 **teaspoon organic lemon zest**

1 **tablespoon (16 g) tamarind paste (optional)**

1 **pound (455 g) small fish (such as sardines or anchovies), heads on, roughly chopped**

In a medium bowl, combine the water, salt, bay leaves, peppercorns, lemon zest, and tamarind paste. Pack the fish into a large fermenting jar and press down firmly. Pour the brine mixture over all, adding more brine, if necessary, to cover 1 inch (2.5 cm) above the fish. Cap the jar tightly and leave in a dark spot at room temperature for 7 to 10 days. Give the jar a shake every few days. Pour the contents into a fine-mesh strainer over a large bowl, collecting the liquid and discarding the solids. Store the fish sauce in the refrigerator, where it will keep for up to 1 week.

Yield: About 2 cups (475 ml)

Note Use in Thai and other Asian dishes that call for fish sauce or use in place of soy sauce. Add fish sauce to any heated soup instead of salt. It's particularly tasty with coconut curries that include cilantro.

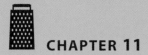

CHAPTER 11

Condiments and Relishes

Eating live cultured condiments and relishes are an ideal way to incorporate fermented foods into your daily fare. Whether it's fermented ketchup, mustard, or mayonnaise added to sandwiches, chips, or spread over meats, fish, or rice dishes, these are easy to make and easier to use.

Digestive Orange, Ginger, and Raisin Relish

Aside from the interesting flavor, the combination of ginger and oranges can spice up your overall wellness. Filled with prebiotic fiber and packed with essential nutrients and rejuvenating compounds, this relish contains tons of anti-inflammatory vitamin C and antioxidants.

3   cups (495 g) peeled, roughly chopped oranges

1   tablespoon (6 g) grated orange zest

½   cup (75 g) raisins

   Zest of 1 medium lemon

½   cup (170 g) unrefined sweetener (rapadura, raw honey, maple syrup)

¼   cup (25 g) chopped fresh ginger

¼   teaspoon ground ginger, plus more as desired

1   clove, ground, or ½ teaspoon ground cloves

   Pinch of fine sea salt

¼   cup (60 ml) Easy Whey (page 92)

Place the oranges, orange zest, raisins, lemon zest, sweetener, fresh and ground ginger, clove, salt, and whey in the bowl of a food processor and process until finely chopped. Transfer the mixture to a 1-quart (946-ml) fermenting jar, leaving 1 inch (2.5 cm) of space below the jar rim. Cover tightly with a lid or an airlock. Set in a dark place at room temperature for 2 to 3 days. Transfer to the refrigerator, where it will keep for up to 3 weeks.

Yield: About 3 cups (735 g)

Cleansing Beet and Apple Relish ▶

The sweet beets in this relish marry deliciously with the tart apples, while the ginger adds a tangy, pungent taste. Beets help cleanse toxins from your body by boosting liver function, and apples contain fiber and restore digestive function. Fermenting this combo increases their cleansing and detoxifying effects in addition to their probiotics.

3   large apples, cored, with peels left on

3   large beets, peeled

½   cup (80 g) chopped red onion

½   teaspoon grated fresh ginger

1   tablespoon (18 g) fine sea salt

¼   cup (60 ml) Easy Whey (page 92)

3   or 4 whole cloves

Place the apples, beets, onion, ginger, salt, and whey in the bowl of a food processor. Process until finely minced. Transfer the mixture to a 1-quart (946-ml) fermenting jar; add the cloves, and press down until brine covers the fruits and vegetables. Cap tightly and ferment at room temperature for 5 to 7 days. Remove the cloves. Transfer the jar to the refrigerator, where the relish will keep for up to 6 weeks.

Yield: About 1 quart (980 g)

Note Beets are available year-round, so you can have this tasty relish any time to top pancakes or omelets, or to serve with grilled or baked meats and fish.

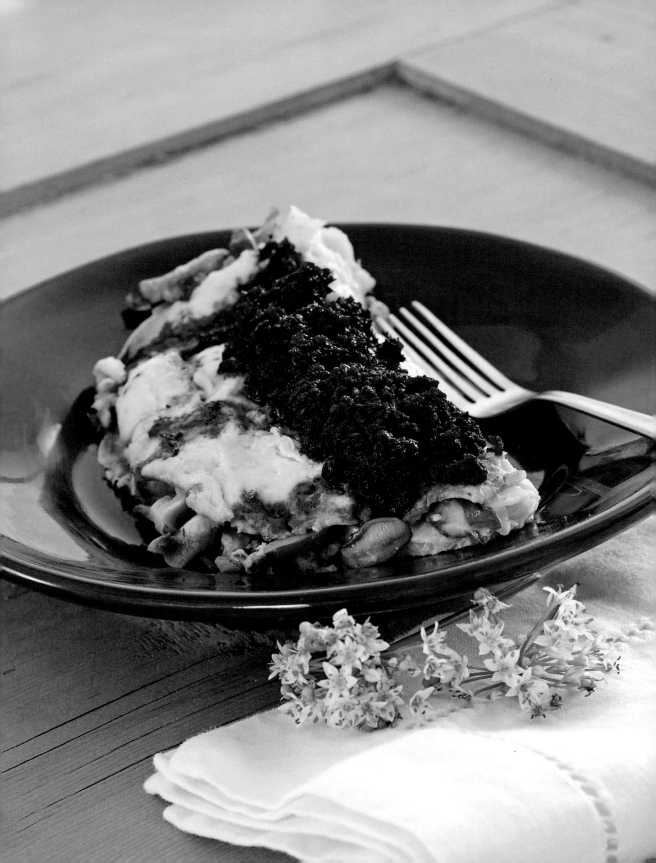

Heart-Healthy Mayonnaise

This highly nutritious and yummy mayonnaise is high in vitamin E, which helps the heart and lungs function properly, as well as aids in blood circulation.

3 egg yolks

1 teaspoon Dijon mustard, or ½ teaspoon dry mustard

1 tablespoon (15 ml) lemon juice

½ teaspoon fine sea salt

2 tablespoons (30 ml) Easy Whey (page 92)

1 cup (235 ml) extra-virgin olive oil

1 to 2 tablespoons (4–8 g) chopped fresh dill or tarragon

Allow all ingredients to come to room temperature. Place the egg yolks, mustard, lemon juice, salt, and whey in the bowl of a food processor and process until smooth. With the motor running, drizzle in the olive oil, a few drops at a time, until all is added. Remove the mixture from the food processor and stir in the dill or tarragon. Spoon the mixture into a 1-pint (473-ml) fermenting jar and cover tightly with a lid. Ferment at room temperature for 8 to 12 hours. Transfer the jar to the refrigerator, where the mayonnaise will keep for up to 8 weeks.

Yield: About 1½ cups (340 g)

Anticancer Beetroot-Horseradish Relish

Beets have been known to slow the growth of tumors in cancer patients. Horseradish has known antibiotic properties and is one of the few vegetables for which processing actually improves its anticancer benefits. Together, these benefits are greatly enhanced through fermentation.

6 medium beets, washed and trimmed

¼ pound (115 g) horseradish, peeled and chopped

2 tablespoons (36 g) fine sea salt

¼ cup (60 ml) Easy Whey (page 92)

Preheat the oven to 300°F (150°C, or gas mark 2). Place the beets in a baking dish, and bake for 45 minutes. Cool to room temperature before peeling and coarsely chopping the beets. Place the beets, horseradish, salt, and whey in the bowl of a food processor and process until smoother but still chunky. Spoon the mixture into a 1-pint (473-ml) fermenting jar and cover tightly with a lid; ferment at room temperature for 3 days. Transfer the jar to the refrigerator, where the relish will keep for up to 2 months.

Yield: About 1 pint (490 g)

Note Horseradish contains up to ten times the amount of cancer-fighting compounds, called glucosinolates, than any other vegetable that contains them.

Must-Have Honey-Dill Mustard*

Enjoy the spicy, pungent taste of fermented mustard naturally sweetened with honey.

½ **cup (120 ml) filtered water**

3 **tablespoons (12 g) chopped fresh dill, or 3 tablespoons (9 g) dried**

3 **tablespoons (45 ml) Easy Whey (page 92)**

¼ **cup (85 g) locally harvested raw honey**

2 **teaspoons fine sea salt**

1 **cup (144 g) dry mustard**

1 **tablespoon (11 g) whole mustard seed, crushed (optional)**

In a small bowl, add the water, dill, whey, honey, salt, dry mustard, and mustard seed and mix well. Pour the mixture into a 1-pint (473-ml) fermenting jar, leaving at least 1 inch (2.5 cm) of space below the top of the jar. Cap tightly and allow the mustard to ferment for 3 to 5 days. Transfer the jar to the refrigerator, where the mustard will keep for a couple of months.

Yield: 1½ cups (264 g)

✳ See image on page 179

> *Note A great choice for those watching their weight, mustard has the capacity to increase the body's metabolic rate as well as ease the process of digestion.*

Infection-Fighting Fermented Chili Sauce*

The amazing health-promoting compounds present in both fresh chile peppers and garlic are at their most potent when you ferment them. Chiles are packed with vitamins A and C, beta-carotene, and other antioxidants that fight infection, while garlic is a natural antibiotic in its own right. Spice up your diet and live longer with this sauce.

1 **cup (144 g) chopped chile peppers**

4 **cloves garlic, peeled and minced**

1 **teaspoon chopped ginger**

1 **teaspoon locally harvested raw honey**

1 **teaspoon fine sea salt**

¼ **cup (60 ml) Easy Whey (page 92)**

Place the chiles, garlic, ginger, honey, salt, and whey in the bowl of a food processor and process until smooth. Spoon the mixture into a 1-quart (946-ml) fermenting jar and cover loosely with a lid. Ferment at room temperature for 5 to 6 days. Transfer the jar to the refrigerator, where the chili sauce will keep for several months.

Yield: About 1 quart (1100 g)

✳ See image on page 179

> *Note Add this sauce to stir-fries or curries, or use it in soups, on pizzas, and in a variety of dishes featuring meat, fish, and chicken.*

Prebiotic Rhubarb-Ginger Relish

Tart and tasty, rhubarb is known for its astringent powers and ability to promote detoxification. It is a natural laxative and is loaded with wonderful prebiotic fiber.

3½ cups (350 g) coarsely chopped rhubarb, rinsed

    Zest of 1 small lemon

⅔ cup (230 g) unrefined sweetener (rapadura, raw honey, maple syrup)

½ cup (120 g) coarsely chopped crystallized ginger

1 teaspoon finely chopped ginger

¼ teaspoon ground nutmeg

    Dash of sea salt

¼ cup (60 ml) Easy Whey (page 92)

Place the rhubarb, lemon zest, sweetener, gingers, nutmeg, salt, and whey in the bowl of a food processor and process until finely chopped. Transfer the mixture to a 1-quart (946-ml) fermenting jar, leaving 1 inch (2.5 cm) free space below the jar rim. Cover tightly with a lid and ferment at room temperature for 2 to 3 days. Transfer the jar to the refrigerator, where the relish will keep for a few weeks.

Yield: About 3 cups (735 g)

Note Spread this lively relish on sourdough sandwiches, or over meat and fish dishes.

Bone-Building Ketchup

Here's a tangy, spicy, and sweet tomato ketchup you'll love. Tomatoes are high in antioxidants and especially rich in lycopene, which are important for bone health. Enhance the flavor of foods while adding healthy probiotics.

1½ cups (390 g) tomato paste

3 tablespoons (60 g) locally harvested raw honey

1 tablespoon (10 g) chopped onion

1 clove garlic, chopped

¼ cup (60 ml) Easy Whey (page 92)

¼ teaspoon cayenne pepper

3 tablespoons (45 ml) raw apple cider vinegar

1 teaspoon fine sea salt

In a small bowl, mix together the tomato paste, honey, onion, garlic, whey, cayenne, vinegar, and salt. Transfer the mixture to a 1-pint (473-ml) fermenting jar, leaving 1 inch (2.5 cm) free space below the jar rim. Cover loosely with a cloth or lid. Ferment at room temperature for 2 to 3 days. Transfer the jar to the refrigerator, where the ketchup will keep for a few weeks.

Yield: About 1½ cups (360 g)

Note If you're using canned tomatoes, choose organic because they have a higher lycopene content than non-organic brands.

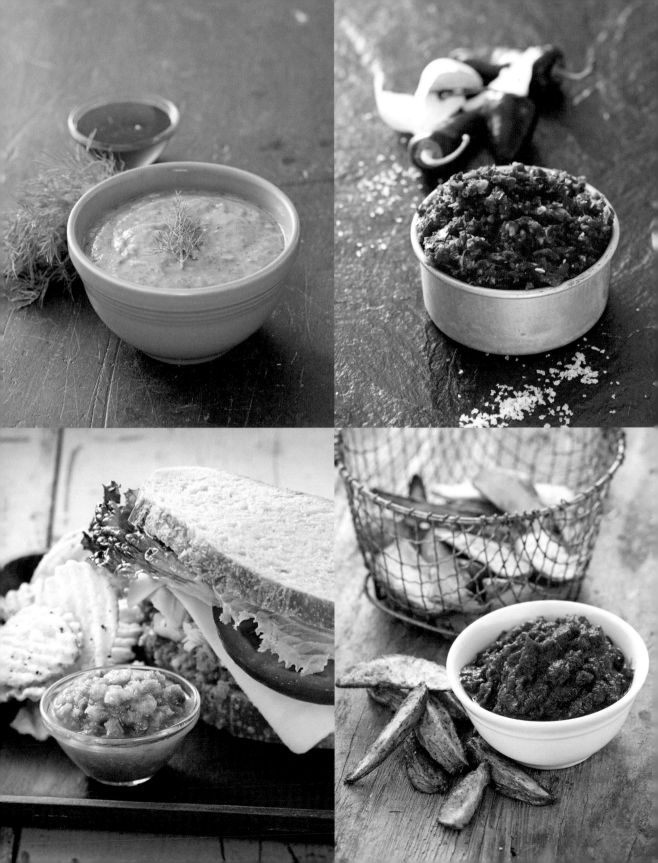

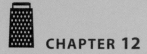

CHAPTER 12

Probiotic Beverages and Tonics

The probiotic beverages and tonics in this section are both nourishing and strengthening to your immune system. They are packed with vitamins and minerals and are a delicious yet inexpensive way to restore and maintain digestive health and to bring your whole body back into balance. They differ from the sweet, sugary beverages that you may be used to; these tonics and beverages are tangy, fizzy, mildly sweet, and sometimes sour, and are teeming with enzymes and friendly microorganisms that help balance your inner ecosystem.

Kombucha tea is a sweetened tea fermented from a symbiotic culture of bacteria and yeast, called a "SCOBY" for short. The SCOBY is sometimes called the "mother" or the "mushroom," although it is not a mushroom at all, mainly because the microorganisms exist in a tough, layered, mush-roomlike shape. The organisms feed on the sugar in the brewed tea, causing the living SCOBY to develop a fresh light-colored layer on top. You can purchase a SCOBY, or you can cultivate your own, which is probably the easiest way when you are starting out. The size does not really matter because smaller ones will ferment a new batch of prepared tea as well as larger ones. You'll find sellers in the Resources section. Kombucha contains enzymes, amino acids, and polyphenols, all produced by these beneficial microorganisms.

Refreshing Kombucha Tea

Tart, refreshing, and slightly effervescent, kombucha is a fermented beverage with a taste similar to that of apple cider. It contains beneficial yeast and bacteria that will help reestablish healthy gut bacteria. During fermentation, the yeast and bacteria feed on the sugar and get the fermentation process going. As a result, the finished product does not contain much sugar or caffeine.

2 to 3 teaspoons (3.2–4.8 g) black or green tea (or a combination), or 2 or 3 tea bags

1 quart (946 ml) boiling filtered water

3 tablespoons (39 g) unrefined sugar

½ to 1 cup (120–235 ml) kombucha tea, from a previous batch or store-bought (this is called backslopping)

1 kombucha SCOBY starter culture (see Resources)

Place the tea in a heat-proof glass container and add the boiling water. Let steep for at least 15 minutes, or longer, depending on how strong you like your tea. Strain the tea into a glass brewing container with a wide mouth. Add the sugar and stir until dissolved. Allow the tea to cool to a drinkable temperature.

Add the reserved kombucha tea, and then place the SCOBY into the liquid. Cover with a clean towel, ensuring that the cloth does not touch the SCOBY, and secure with a rubber band. Store in a warm place, away from direct sunlight, for 7 to 10 days. Brewing time will vary, depending on room temperature: the warmer the temperature, the shorter the brewing time.

Remove the SCOBY. The finished kombucha tea should be pleasantly tangy. If the tea is still sweet, it has not fermented long enough. If the tea is very tart and vinegary, it has brewed for too long. Do some taste tests and experiment to find out how you prefer your tea, and then brew it to your taste. Store kombucha tea in a tightly capped glass container in the cupboard or in the refrigerator. Store the kombucha SCOBY in a bowl covered with a cloth. Do not store it in the refrigerator.

Yield: 1 quart (946 ml)

Note *If you are just starting out, you will need to get a kombucha starter kit (see Resources). The kombucha tea will often grow little SCOBYs on top of the liquid during storage. This is normal and nothing to be concerned about. Scoop them out or simply avoid them when you drink your kombucha. SCOBYs need plenty of oxygen to start fermentation, so choose storage containers that are wider than they are high.*

Revitalizing Rejuvelac

Rejuvelac is a probiotic tonic used to replenish microflora and help rebuild digestion. It is slightly fizzy with a subtle sweetness and lemony flavor. It contains vitamins B complex, E, and K and is rich in enzymes. Use rejuvelac instead of water in smoothies, and drink it in between meals to cleanse your colon.

1 cup (98 g) wheat berries or other whole grains

1 quart (946 ml) filtered water

Dash of raw apple cider vinegar

Soak the grains overnight in warm nonchlorinated water. Drain and rinse well. Transfer to a sprouting device or tray suitable for sprouting (plastic kitty-litter trays work well). Allow the grains to sit for 2 to 3 days, and drain, rinse, and stir the grains each day until they sprout. A small tail should appear. Once your grains sprout, rinse them well and transfer them to a mason jar. Cover with the 1 quart (946 ml) water, add a dash of vinegar, and let it sit for 2 to 3 days. Expect some bubbling. The rejuvelac is ready when it appears cloudy and smells pleasantly sour. Pour the contents into a fine-mesh strainer over a large bowl. Discard the grain and store the liquid in a clean, tightly sealed jar. Transfer the jar to the refrigerator, where the tonic will keep for up to 2 weeks.

Yield: 1 quart (946 ml)

Note Traditional rejuvelac is made from whole wheat grains, called berries, but it can be made using whole rye, oats, barley, millet, rice, or buckwheat grains.

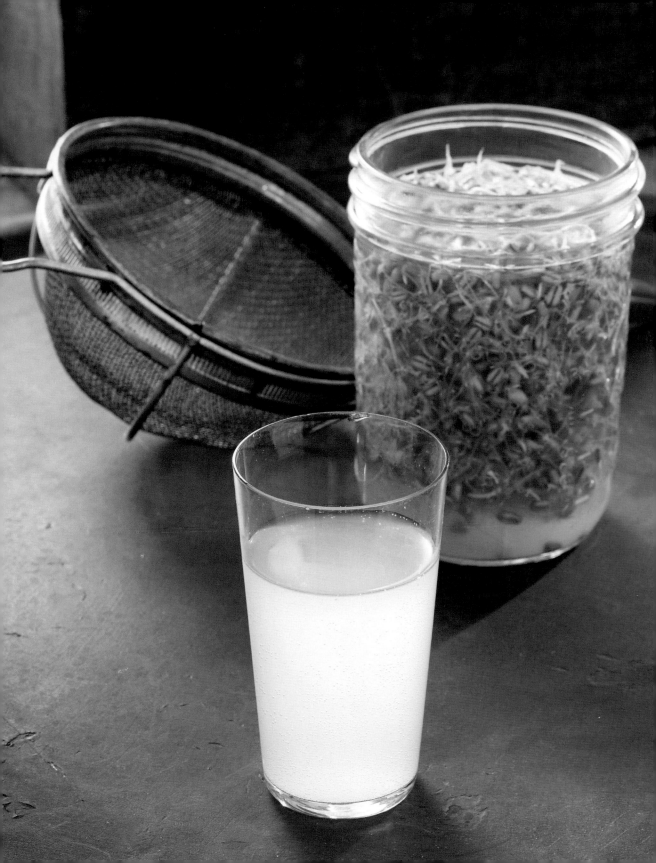

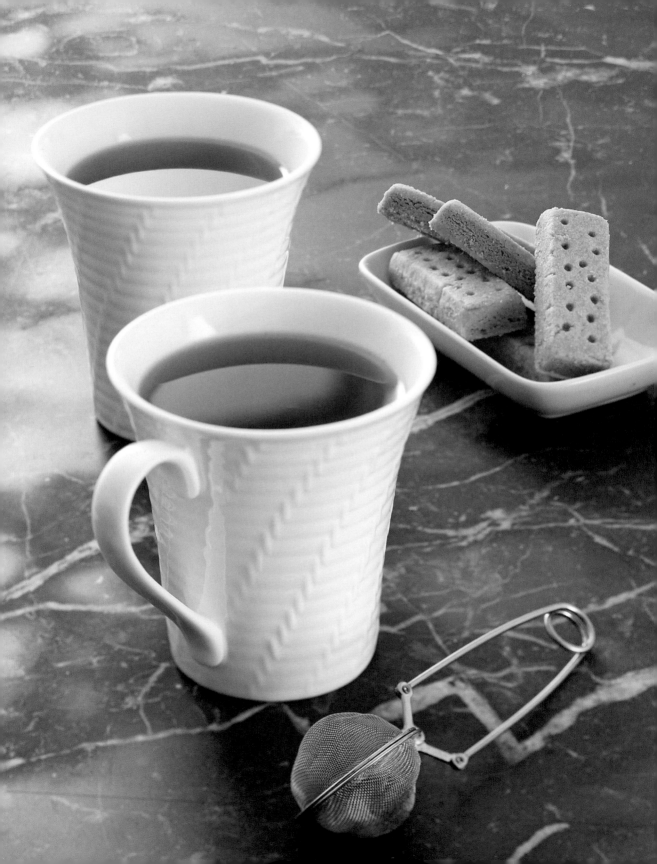

Energizing Green Tea Kombucha

You can count on having increased energy and stamina from drinking kombucha tea, and this is enhanced when you make it with green tea. Some athletes have reported more endurance and reduced muscle aches, pain, and fatigue from this amazing elixir.

6 green tea bags

¾ cup (255 g) unrefined sweetener (rapadura, raw honey, maple syrup)

3½ quarts (3.5 L) filtered water, divided, plus additional as needed

1 kombucha SCOBY starter culture (see Resources)

1½ cups (355 ml) finished kombucha (homemade or store-bought)

Combine the tea bags, sweetener, and 3 cups (705 ml) of the water in a 3-quart (3-L) pot and bring to a boil; remove from the heat and cover. Let steep for 15 minutes; remove the tea bags and squeeze the liquid out of them.

Add 2 quarts (2 L) of the cool water to the pot, then pour the cooled tea into a gallon (4-L) jar. Add the SCOBY and finished kombucha. Add enough water to fill the jar up to the shoulder. Cover the jar with a clean cloth, taking care that it doesn't touch the SCOBY. Let it sit at room temperature for 5 to 10 days, or until it's bubbly and mildly sweet and sour tasting.

Pour the finished kombucha into another gallon container, leaving the SCOBY and 1½ cups (355 ml) of kombucha behind (this can be used to make more batches). Pour the finished kombucha into jars and cap tightly. Let sit at room temperature for 1 to 2 days to build up carbonation, then chill until ready to serve. Kombucha keeps indefinitely and becomes more sour and vinegary with age.

Yield: 3 quarts (3 L)

The earliest record of kombucha seems to date from 414 BCE in Korea. In China, it showed up in 221 BCE, during the Tsin Dynasty, and later found its way to Japan, Russia, and India.

Note Always use a sweetener when making your kombucha because this is what your starter culture uses for food, and without it, it cannot proliferate or make a probiotic beverage.

Digestive Lemon-Ginger Kombucha

Increase the medicinally rich nutritive properties already present in kombucha by adding herbs and spices. Do so once you have made a few batches of plain kombucha tea. This brew's addition of ginger makes it particularly pleasing to the digestive system.

6 **green tea bags**

¾ **cup (255 g) unrefined sweetener (rapadura, raw honey, maple syrup)**

1 **teaspoon organic lemon zest**

1 **teaspoon grated ginger**

3½ **quarts (3.5 L) filtered water, divided, plus additional as needed**

1 **kombucha SCOBY starter culture (see Resources)**

1½ **cups (355 ml) finished kombucha, store-bought or homemade (page 185)**

Combine the tea bags, sweetener, lemon zest, ginger, and 3 cups (705 ml) of the water in a 3-quart (3-L) pot and bring to a boil; remove from the heat and cover. Let steep for 15 minutes. Remove the tea bags and squeeze the liquid out of them.

Add 2 quarts (2 L) of the cool water to the pot, then pour the cooled tea into a gallon (4-L) jar. Add the SCOBY and finished kombucha, then add enough water to fill the jar up to 3 inches (7.5 cm) below the rim. Cover with a clean cloth, taking care that it doesn't touch the SCOBY. Let sit at room temperature for 5 to 10 days, or until it's bubbly and has a slightly sweet and sour taste.

Pour the finished kombucha into another gallon container, leaving the SCOBY and 1½ cups (355 ml) of kombucha behind (this can be used to make more batches). Pour the finished kombucha into jars and cap tightly. Let sit at room temperature for 1 to 2 days to build up carbonation, then chill until ready to serve. Kombucha keeps indefinitely and becomes more sour and vinegary with age.

Yield: 3 quarts (3 L)

Note Avoid using teas with aromatic oils—such as Earl Grey, which is made with bergamot citrus oil—because the oils can kill your kombucha. Depending on the environment and conditions in which it is brewed, kombucha can become infected with a variety of other microorganisms. Normally, the acidity of kombucha protects against unfriendly pathogens; however, if you suffer any negative symptoms when drinking it, there is a small possibility that your brew has been infected. An unpleasant smell or taste is a tell-tale sign.

Blood-Purifying Beet Kvass

Kvass is a probiotic drink that's been consumed in Eastern Europe since ancient times. This version uses beets, which are wonderful for purifying the blood and cleansing the liver. They're also loaded with electrolytes and vitamin C, and fermenting them only enhances their nutritive properties.

6 medium (or 4 large) organic beets, peeled and coarsely chopped

½ cup (120 ml) Easy Whey (page 92)

2 tablespoons (36 g) fine sea salt

1 organic lemon, halved (optional)

1 teaspoon chopped ginger (optional)

1 quart (946 ml) filtered water

Place the beets, whey, salt, lemon, and ginger in a 1-quart (946-ml) jar, leaving 1 inch (2.5 cm) free space below the jar rim. Pour in the water. Allow the covered kvass to ferment at room temperature for 2 to 3 days. Pour the contents into a fine-mesh strainer over a large bowl, reserving the liquid. The beets can be saved for your next batch. The liquid should be somewhat thick and slightly bubbly. Pour the kvass into a jar and refrigerate. Kvass will keep in the refrigerator for up to 2 months or possibly longer.

Yield: 1 quart (946 ml)

Note *The word kvass is derived from Old Eastern Slavic and means "yeast" or "leaven" because it was commonly made from black or regular rye bread. Use the discarded beets from this version in borscht, a traditional Russian soup legendary among centenarians!*

Hydrating Coconut Water

High in electrolytes and enzymes, coconut water is the liquid found in the center of the coconut. It has a very light consistency and contains a good composition of minerals, such as calcium, magnesium, iron, manganese, and zinc, along with B-complex and C vitamins that hydrate and refresh cells. The addition of kefir grains makes these nutrients more available to the body while adding beneficial flora.

1 **medium to large young green drinking coconut**

1 **tablespoon (30 g) hydrated water kefir grains (See Resources, page 204)**

Using a sharp knife, carefully chisel a hole in the shell of the coconut. Tilt the coconut and carefully pour the coconut water into a wide-mouth 1-quart (946-ml) jar. Add the kefir grains. Cover the jar with a lid or an airlock, and let sit at room temperature for 24 hours. Scoop out the grains and add them to a new batch of coconut water, or store them in some milk or water in the refrigerator for later use. Refrigerate the coconut water until ready to serve. It will keep for up to 3 months.

Yield: About 2 cups (475 ml)

> *Note* *Fresh, tender coconuts can be stored at room temperature for 5 to 10 days prior to opening. Use coconut water in smoothies and desserts, to cook rice, or to add to soups and marinades.*

Wild Honey Mead ▶

Known as honey wine, mead has been renowned for centuries as an aphrodisiac that originated in ancient Europe. Honey is a natural energy booster and immune system builder that contains a large amount of friendly bacteria: six species of Lactobacilli *and four species of* Bifidobacteria.

1 **quart (946 ml) filtered water**

1 **cup (245 g) locally harvested raw honey**

1 **tablespoon (6 g) whole cloves**

In a medium saucepan over medium-high heat, bring the water to a boil. Add the honey. Turn off the heat and stir well. Add the cloves and let stand, covered with a clean cloth, until cool. Transfer to a 1-quart (946-ml) glass jar and cover with a lid. Place in a cool, dark place to ferment for 14 to 16 days. Transfer to a fermentation jar with an airlock and ferment an additional 2 to 3 weeks. Periodically test the flavor and alcohol content level until satisfied, then refrigerate. Mead will keep indefinitely.

Yield: 1 quart (946 ml)

> *Note* *The word "honeymoon" is believed to be derived from the ancient European custom of having newlyweds drink honey wine for a whole moon cycle (month) to increase their fertility and chances of getting pregnant.*

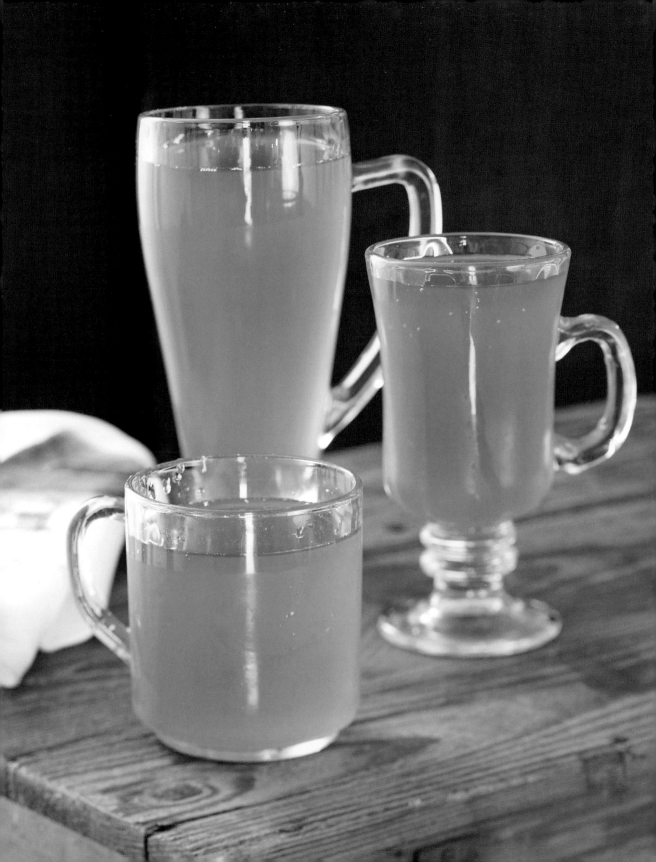

Cleansing Probiotic Limonade

If you like fruit juice, then you'll like this even better. Add a healthy dose of probiotics to refreshing limonade that the whole family will enjoy. It's loaded with antioxidants, especially vitamin C; alkalinizes your system to enhance cleansing; and revs up your metabolism.

¾ **cup (175 ml) sucanat or evaporated cane juice (lightly refined sweetener)**

2 **quarts (2 L) filtered water, divided**

Juice of 5 lemons

Juice of 5 limes

1 **cup (235 ml) Easy Whey (page 92)**

In a large pot over medium heat, dissolve the sugar in 2 cups (475 ml) of the water. Remove from the heat and add the remaining 1½ quarts (1420 ml) cool water. Pour the sugar water into a gallon (4-L) jar. Allow it to cool to room temperature. Add the lemon juice, lime juice, and whey. Add enough water to fill within 1 inch (2.5 cm) of the top of the jar. Cover with a lid or an airlock. Let sit at room temperature for 2 to 3 days, or until the sweetness is reduced to your desired taste. Transfer the jar to the refrigerator and chill the limonade thoroughly before serving. This keeps indefinitely, but the sweetness reduces over time.

Yield: About 2 quarts (2 L)

Note Be careful when you open the airlock bottles because the contents are highly carbonated and can explosively overflow.

Fermented Virgin Mary with a Twist ▶

Thanks to the antioxidants lycopene and vitamin C it contains, this delicious cocktail can help prevent free radicals from ever reaching the cells, thereby reducing your chances of cancer. The high potassium and mineral content give it cardioprotective properties, which are made more potent by fermentation. It's refreshing and nourishing.

6 **medium Roma tomatoes, quartered**

¼ **medium onion**

½ **medium cucumber, peeled**

¼ **bell pepper, seeded**

½ **chile pepper, seeded**

1 **clove garlic**

Juice of ½ lemon

½ **tablespoon (9 g) fine sea salt**

3 **tablespoons (45 ml) Easy Whey (page 92)**

Place the tomatoes, onion, cucumber, bell pepper, chile pepper, and garlic into a juicer and extract the juice. Pour the juice into a wide-mouth 1-quart (946-ml) jar. Add the lemon juice, salt, and whey, and whisk together. Ensure there's at least 1 inch (2.5 cm) of room at the top of the jar, then cover with a lid or an airlock. Let sit at room temperature for 12 hours or overnight. Transfer the jar to the refrigerator for 2 to 3 hours. Mix again before serving. This drink will keep for a week or two, but it's best drunk within a few days.

Yield: About 2 cups (475 ml)

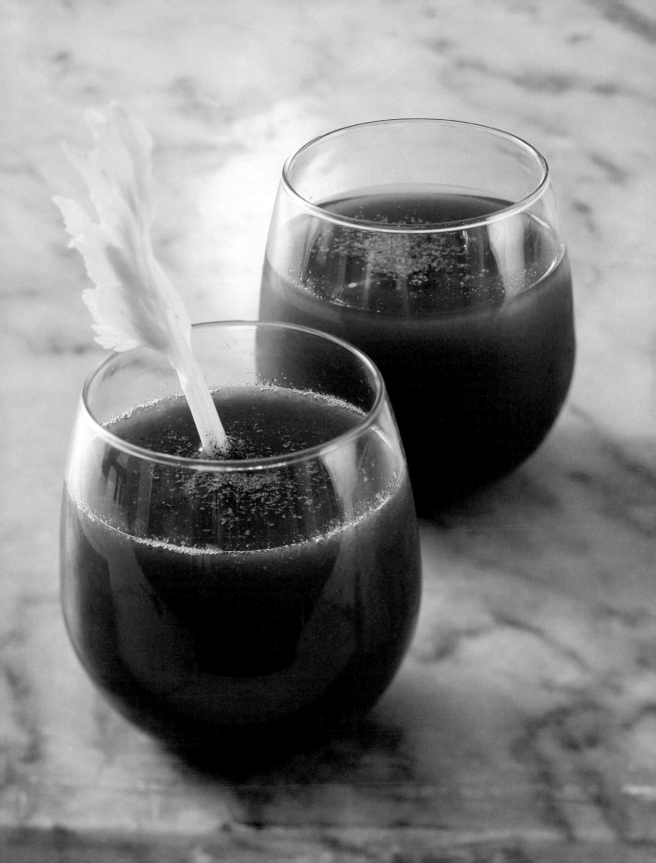

References

CHAPTER 1

Ackerman, Jennifer. 2012. How bacteria in our bodies protect our health. *Scientific American* (May).

Adams, M. 1990. Topical aspects of fermented foods. *Trends in Food Science & Technology* 1:141–144.

Anthony, D. H., and E. M. Frank. 1989. Prophylactic and therapeutic aspects of fermented milk. *Am J Clin Nutri* 49 (4): 675–684.

Beuchat, L. R. 2012. 13 indigenous fermented foods. www.wiley-vch.de/books/biotech/pdf/v09indig.pdf.

Campbell-McBride, N. 2010. *Gut and psychology syndrome: Natural treatment for autism, dyspraxia, A.D.D., dyslexia, A.D.H.D., depression, schizophrenia.* Cambridge, UK: Medinform Publishing.

Cecilia R., M. Marta, et al. 2010.Therapeutic effect of *Streptococcus thermophilus* CRL1190-fermented milk on chronic gastritis. *World J Gastroenterol* 16 (13): 1622–1630.

Chen Jian Liu, Fu Ming Gong, et al. 2012. Natural populations of lactic acid bacteria in douchi from Yunan province, China. *Biomed & Biotechnol* 13 (4): 298–306.

Emilia, H., B. Alojz B, et al. 2011. Prebiotics and bioactive natural substances induce changes of composition and metabolic activities of the colonic microflora in cancerous rats. *ACTA* 59 (2): 271–274.

Fabian, J. C., J. L. Sandrine, et al. 2012. Milk fermented by *Propionibacterium freudenreichii* induces apoptosis of HGT-1 human gastric cancer cells. *Plos ONE* 7(3): e31892. doi:10:1371/journal. pone.0031892.

Fermented fruits and vegetables. A global perspective. Introduction. FAO Corporate Document Repository. www.fao.org/docrep/x0560e/x0560e05.htm.

Gershon, M. 1999. *The second brain: A groundbreaking new understanding of nervous disorders of the stomach and intestine.* New York: Harper Perennial.

Giongo, A., K. A. Gano, et al. 2011. Toward defining the autoimmune microbiome for type 1 diabetes. *ISME J* 5:82–91.

Goossens, H., M. Ferech, R. Vander Stichele, and M. Elseviers, ESAC ProjectGroup. 2005. Outpatient antibiotic use in Europe and association with resistance: A cross-national database study. *Lancet* 365:579–587.

Gregor, M. F., and G. S. Hotamisligil. 2011. Inflammatory mechanisms in obesity. *Annu Rev Immunol* 29:415–445.

Lawrence, R. 2007. *Fermentation and Its Health Benefits. Transform Your Health.* www.transformyourhealth.com/webnewsletters/oct07/fermentationhealthbenefitsarticle.htm.

Lee, Y. K., and S. K. Mazmanian. 2010. Has the microbiota played a critical role in the evolution of the adaptive immune system? *Science* 330:1768–1773.

Ley, R. E., F. Bäckhed, et al. 2005. Obesity alters gut microbial ecology. *Proc Natl Acad Sci USA* 102:11070–11075.

Ljungh, A., and T. Wadstrom, eds. 2009. Lactobacillus *molecular biology: From genomics to probiotics.* Lund University, Faculty of Medicine, Lund, Sweden: Caister Academic Press.

Sahlin, Peter. 1999. *Fermentation as a method of food processing.* Lund Institute of Technology, Dept. Food Chemistry (May).

Sommer, M.O., G. Dantas, and G. M. Church. 2009. Functional characterization of the antibiotic resistance reservoir in the human microflora. *Science* 325:1128–1131.

Steinkraus, K. H. 1983. *Handbook of indigenous fermented foods.* New York: Marcel Dekker.

------. 1996. *Handbook of indigenous fermented foods*, 2nd ed. New York: Marcel Dekker.

Tannock, Gerald W., ed. 2005. *Probiotics and prebiotics: Scientific analysis.* Wyndmondham, UK: Caister Academic Press.

------. 2006. Probiotics: A critical review. *Journal of Clinical Gastroenterology* 40 (5): 458.

Turnbaugh, P. J., V. K. Ridaura, et al., 2009. The effect of diet on the human gut microbiome: A metagenomic analysis in humanized gnotobiotic mice. *Sci Transl Med* 1:6–14.

Wen, L., R. E. Ley, et al. 2008. Innate immunity and intestinal microbiota in the development of type 1 diabetes. *Nature* 455:1109–1113.

Willyard, Cassandra. 2011. Microbiome: Gut reaction. *Nature: International Weekly Journal of Science* 479:S5–S7.

Wu, G. D., J. Chen, et al. 2011. Linking long-term dietary patterns with gut microbial enterotypes. *Science* 334:105–108.

CHAPTER 2

Anthony, D. H., and E. M. Frank. 1989. Prophylactic and therapeutic aspects of fermented milk. *Am J Clin Nutri* 49:675–684.

Campbell-McBride, N. 2010. *Gut and psychology syndrome: Natural treatment for autism, dyspraxia, A.D.D., dyslexia, A.D.H.D., depression, schizophrenia.* Cambridge, UK: Medinform Publishing.

Cecilia, R., M. Marta, et al. 2010. Therapeutic effect of *Streptococcus thermophilus* CRL1190-fermented milk on chronic gastritis. *World J Gastroenterol* 16 (13): 1622–1630.

Chen Jian Liu, Fu Ming Gong, et al. 2012. Natural populations of lactic acid bacteria in douchi from Yunan province, China. *Biomed & Biotechnol* 13 (4): 298–306.

Emilia, H., B. Alojz B, et al. 2011 Prebiotics and bioactive natural substances induce changes of composition and metabolic activities of the colonic microflora in cancerous rats. *Acta biochim Pol* 59 (2): 271–274.

Fabian, J. C., J. L. Sandrine, et al. 2012. Milk fermented by *Propionibacterium freudenreichii* induces apoptosis of HGT-1 human gastric cancer cells. *Plos ONE* 7 (3): e31892. doi:10:1371/journal.pone.0031892.

Fallon, S., and M. G. Enig. 2001. *Nourishing traditions: The cookbook that challenges politically correct nutrition and the diet dictocrats,* 2nd ed. Washington, DC: NewTrends Publishing.

Goossens, H., M. Ferech, R. Vander Stichele, and M. Elseviers, ESAC ProjectGroup. 2005. Outpatient antibiotic use in Europe and association with resistance: A cross-national database study. *Lancet* 365:579–587.

Jie, Y., S. Zhihong, et al. 2009 Rapid identification of lactic acid bacteria isolated from homemade fermented milk in Tibet. *J Gen Appl Microbiol* 55:181–190.

Margaret, C. M., C. L. Eric, et al. 1991. Strains and species of lactic acid bacteria in fermented milks (yoghurts): Effect on in vivo lactose tolerance. *Am J Clin Nutr* 54:1041–1046.

Merenstein, D., M. Murphy, et al. 2010. Use of a fermented dairy probiotic drink containing *Lactobacillus casei* (DN-114 001) to decrease the rate of illness in kids: The DRINK study, a patient-oriented, double-blind, cluster-randomized, placebo-controlled, clinical trial. *European Journal of Clinical Nutrition* 64:669–677.

Merit, M. T., C. Ania, et al. 2009. Effect of the consumption of a fermented dairy product containing *Bifidobacterium lactis* DN-173 010 on constipation in childhood: A multicentre randomised controlled trial (NTRTC: 1571). *BMC Pediatrics* 9:22. doi:10.1186/1471-2431-922.

Molis, C., B. Flourie, F. Ouarne, et al. 1996. Digestion, excretion, and energy value of fructooligosaccharides in healthy humans. *Am J Clin Nutr* 64:324–328.

Parvez, S., K. Malik, A. Kang, H. Kim. 2006. Review article: Probiotics and their fermented food products are beneficial for health. *The Society for Applied Microbiology, Journal of Applied Microbiology* 100:1171–1185.

Pierre, M. K. F. Z. Ngoufack, M. Félicité, Morsi EL-SODA, L. C. Muhammad. 2012. Antimicrobial and safety properties of *Lactobacilli* isolated from two Cameroonian traditional fermented foods. *Sci Pharm* 80:189–203.

Roberfroid, M. 1993. Dietary fibre, inulin and oligofructose. A review comparing their physiological effects. *Crit Rev Food Sci Nutr* 33:103–148.

------:.2007. Prebiotics: The concept revisited. *J Nutr Suppl.* no. 2, 137: 830S–837S.

Seiji, K, K. Mitsuoki, et al. 2011. Sake lees fermented with lactic acid bacteria prevents allergic rhinitis symptoms and IgE mediated basophil degranulation. *Biochem* 75 (1): 140-144.

Seiko, N., S. Tadashi, et al. 2010. Inhibitory effect of yoghurt on aberrant crypt foci formation in the rat colon and colorectal tumorigenesis in RAS H2 mice. *Exp Anim* 59 (4): 487–494.

Sook , J.R., J.E. Lee, C.H. Lee. 2011. Importance of lactic acid bacteria in Asian fermented foods. *Microbial Cell Fact Suppl* no. 1: S5

Thomas, M., and V. Wieland. 2011. Fermented wheat germ extract—nutritional supplement or anticancer drug? *Nutrition Journal* 10:89. doi:10.1186/1475-2891-10-89.

Toyoaki, W., H. Kazuya, et al. 2009. Oral administration of lactic acid bacteria isolated from traditional South Asian fermented milk "dahi" inhibits the development of atopic dermatitis in Nc/Nga mice. *J Nutri Sci Vitaminol* 55:271–278.

Yoshiaki, M., ITO Chihiro, et al. 2010. Evaluation of flavuglaucin, its derivatives and pyranonigrins produced by molds present in fermented foods for inhibiting tumour promotion. *Biochem* 75 (5P): 1120–1122.

CHAPTER 3

Alberda, C., L. Gramlich, et al. 2007. Effects of probiotic therapy in critically ill patients: A randomized, double-blind, placebo-controlled trial. *Am J Clin Nutr* 85 (3): 816–823.

Bäckhed, F., H. Ding, T. Wang, et al. 2004. The gut microbiota as an environmental factor that regulates fat storage. *Proc Natl Acad Sci U.S.A.* 101 (44): 15718–15723.

Bodera, P., A. Cheialowski. 2008. Immunomodulatory effect of probiotic bacteria. *Recent Patients on Inflammation of Allergy Drug Discovery*. Dept. Biopharmacy, Medical University of Lodz, Poland. 1:90–151.

Bourlioux, P., B. Koletzko, et al. 2003. The intestine and its microflora are partners for the protection of the host: Report on the Danone Symposium "The Intelligent Intestine," held in Paris, June 14, 2002. *Am J Clin Nutri* 78 (4): 675–683.

Campbell-McBride, N. 2010. *Gut and psychology syndrome: Natural treatment for autism, dyspraxia, A.D.D., dyslexia, A.D.H.D., depression, schizophrenia*. Cambridge, UK: Medinform Publishing.

Cani, P. D., J. Amar, M. A. Iglesias, et al. 2007. Metabolic endotoxemia initiates obesity and insulin resistance. *Diabetes* 56:1761–1772.

Chettipalli, N. D., P. Santosh, et al. 2011. Evaluation of the various uses of microorganisms with emphasis on probiotics. *J Microbial Biochem Technol*. doi:10.4172/1948-5948. R1-004.

Clemente, J. C., K. Luke, et al. 2012. The Impact of the gut microbiota on human health: An integrative view. *Recent Patients on Inflammation of Allergy Drug Discovery*. Univ of CO Dept of Chemistry & Biochemistry.

Cunningham-Rundles, S., S. Ahrne, et al. 2000. Probiotics and immune response. *Am J Gastroenterol* 95:S22–S25.

Dong, H., I. Rowland, et al. 2010. Selective effects of *Lactobacillus casei Shirota* on T cell activation, natural killer cell activity and cytokine production. *Clin Exp Immunol* 161 (2): 378–388.

Fabian, J. C., J. L. Sandrine, et al. 2012. Milk fermented by *Propionibacterium freudenreichii* induces apoptosis of HGT-1 human gastric cancer cells. *Plos ONE* 7(3). e31892.doi:10.1371/journal.pone.0031892.

Fang, H., M. Hirotsugar, et al. 2006. *Bifidobacteria* and *Lactobacilli* exhibited different mitogenic activity on murine splenocytes. *Int Journal of Probiotics and Prebiotics* 1 (1): 77–82.

Haard, Norman, et al. 1999. *Fermented cereals: A global perspective*. FAO Agricultural Services Bulletin No. 138. Rome: Food and Agriculture Organization of the United Nations.

Hata, Y., M. Yamamoto, et al. 1996. A placebo-controlled study of the effect of sour milk on blood pressure in hypertensive subjects. *Am J Clin Nutr* 64:767–771.

Hempel, S., et al. 2012. Probiotics for the prevention and treatment of antibiotic-associated diarrhea. A systemic review and meta-analysis. *JAMA* 307 (18): 1959–1969.

Hijova, E., A. Bomba, et al. 2012. Prebiotics and bioactive natural substances induce changes of composition and metabolic activities of the colonic microflora in cancerous rats. *Acta Biochim Pol* 59 (2): 271–274.

Huffnagle, G. B., and S. Wernick. 2007. *The probiotics revolution: The definitive guide to safe, natural health solutions using probiotic and prebiotic foods and supplements*. New York: Bantam Books.

Irvine, S. L., R. Hummelen, et al. 2010. Probiotic yogurt consumption is associated with an increase of CD4 count among people living with HIV/AIDS. *J Clin Gastroenterol* 44 (9): e201–205.

Kalaydjian, A. E., W. Eaton, et al. 2006. The gluten connection: The association between schizophrenia and celiac disease. *Acta Psychiatr Scand* 113 (2): 82–90.

Kathein, J. 2012. Old World fermented foods vital to healthy living and nutritional healing. Béland Organic Foods. Retrieved from http://belandorganicfoods.com/bof/organic-products/kartheins-organic-sauerkraut/fermented-foods.

Kraft, B. D., E. C. Westman, et al. 2009. Schizphrenia, gluten, and low-carbohydrate, ketogenic diets: A case report and review of the literature. *Nutrition & Metabolism* 6:10. doi:10.1186/1743-7075-6-10.

Lawrence, R. 2007. Fermentation and its health benefits. Transform Your Health. Retrieved from www.transformyourhealth.com/webnewsletters/oct07/fermentationhealthbenefitsarticle.htm.

Lee, Y. K., S. Juscilene, et al. 2010. Proinflammatory T-cell responses to gut microbiota promote experimental autoimmune encephalomyelitis. doi:10.1073/PNAS 1000082107.

Ley, R. E., P. J. Turnbaugh, S. Klein, and J. I. Gordon. 2006. Microbial ecology: Human gut microbes associated with obesity. *Nature* 444 (7122): 1022–1023.

Lipsky, E. 1996. *Digestive wellness*. Los Angeles: Keats Publishing.

Lye, H. S., C. Y. Kuan, et al. 2009. The improvement of hypertension by probiotics: Effects on cholesterol, diabetes, rennin, and phytoestrogens. *Int J Mol Sci* 10 (9): 3755–3775.

Margaret, C. M., C. L. Eric, et al. 1991. Strains and species of lactic acid bacteria in fermented milks (yoghurts): Effect on in vivo lactose tolerance. *Am J Clin Nutr* 54:1041–1046.

Marlin, M., P. Verronen, et al. 1997. Dietary therapy with *Lactobacillus* GG, bovine colostrum or bovine immune colostrum in patients with juvenile chronic arthritis: Evaluation of effect on gut defence mechanisms. *Inflammopharmacology* 5 (3): 219–236.

Merenstein, D., M. Murphy, et al. 2010. Use of a fermented dairy probiotic drink containing *Lactobacillus casei* (DN-114 001) to decrease the rate of illness in kids: The DRINK study, a patient-oriented, double-blind, cluster-randomized, placebo-controlled, clinical trial. *European Journal of Clinical Nutrition* 64:669–677.

Musso, G., R. Gambino, et al. 2010. Obesity, diabetes, and gut microbiota: The hygiene hypothesis expanded? *Diabetes Care* 33 (10): 2277–2284.

Palmer, C., E. M. Bik, et al. Development of the human infant intestinal microbiota. *PLoS Biol* 5 (7): e177. doi:10.1371/journal.pbio.0050177.

Parvez, S., K. Malik, A. Kang, H. Kim. 2006. Review article: Probiotics and their fermented food products are beneficial for health. *The Society for Applied Microbiology, Journal of Applied Microbiology* 100:1171–1185.

Peñas, E., et al. 2010. Chemical evaluation and sensory quality of sauerkrauts obtained by natural and induced fermentations at different NaCl levels from *Brassica oleracea* Var. *capitata* Cv. *Bronco* grown in eastern Spain. Effect of storage. *J Agric Food Chem* 58 (6): 3549–3557.

Probiotics help gastric-bypass patients lose weight more quickly. Stanford University News. July 2009. Retrieved from http://news.stanford.edu/news/2009/july8/probiotics-071309.html.

Qin, J., Y. Li, et al. 2012. A metagenome-wide association study of gut microbiota in type 2 diabetes. *Nature*. doi:10.1038/nature11450.

Rajiv, S., S. Saini, et al. 2010. Potential of probiotics in controlling cardiovascular diseases. *J Cardiovasc Dis Res* 1 (4): 213–214.

Ripudaman, S. Beniwal, et al. 2003. A randomized trial of yogurt for prevention of antibiotic-associated diarrhea. *Digestive Diseases and Sciences* 48 (10): 2077–2082.

Roberfroid, M. B. 2000. Prebiotics and probiotics: Are they functional foods? *Am J Clin Nutr* 71:1682S–1687S.

Seiji, K. K. Mitsuoki, et al. 2011. Sake lees fermented with lactic acid bacteria prevents allergic rhinitis symptoms and IgE mediated basophil degranulation. *Biochem* 75 (1): 140-144.

Seiko, N., S. Tadashi, et al. 2010. Inhibitory effect of yoghurt on aberrant crypt foci formation in the rat colon and colorectal tumorigenesis in RAS H2 mice. *Exp Anim* 59 (4): 487–494.

Shurtleff, W., A. Aoyagi. 1976. *The book of miso*. Kanagawa, Japan: Autumn Press.

Sokol, H., B. Pigneur, et al. 2008. *Faecalibacterium prausnitzii* is an anti-inflammatory commensal bacterium identified by gut microbiota analysis of Crohn disease patients. *Proc Natl Acad Sci USA* 105 (43): 16731–16736.

Solga, S. F., G. Buckley, et al. 2008. The effect of a probiotic on hepatic steatosis. *J Clin Gastroenterol* 42:1117–1119.

Steinkraus, K. H. 1983. *Handbook of indigenous fermented foods*. New York: Marcel Dekker.

------. 1996. *Handbook of indigenous fermented foods*, 2nd ed. New York: Marcel Dekker.

Thomas, M., and V. Wieland. 2011. Fermented wheat germ extract—nutritional supplement or anticancer drug? *Nutrition Journal*. doi:10.1186/1475-2891-10-89.

Uronis, J. M., M. Muhlbauer, et al. 2009. Modulation of the intestinal microbiota alters colitis-associated colorectal cancer susceptibility. *PLoS ONE* 4 (6): e6026.

Wang, H. L., D. I. Ruttle, C. W. Hesseltine. 1969. Antibiotic compound from a soybean product fermented by *Rhizopus oligosporus*. *Proc Soc Exp Biol Med* 131:579–583.

Whaling, M. A., I. Luginaah, et al. 2012. Perceptions about probiotic yogurt for health and nutrition in the context of HIV/AIDS in Mwanza, Tanzania. *J Health Popul Nutr* 30 (1): 31–40.

Yoshiaki, M,. I. Chihiro, et al. 2010. Evaluation of flavuglaucin, its derivatives and pyranonigrins produced by molds present in fermented foods for inhibiting tumour promotion. *Biochem* 75 (5P): 1120–1122.

CHAPTER 4

Bohn, L., et al. 2008. Phytate: Impact on environment and human nutrition. A challenge for molecular breeding. *J Zhejiang Univ Sci* B 9 (3): 165–191. www.ncbi.nlm.nih.gov/pmc/articles/PMC2266880.

Dinesh, B. P., R. Bhakyaraj, et al. 2009. A low cost nutritious food "Tempeh"—A review. *World Jour of Dairy & Food Sciences* 4 (1): 22–27.

Egli, I., et al. 2002. The influence of soaking and germination on the phytase activity and phytic acid content of grains and seeds potentially useful for complementary feeding. *Journal of Food Science* 67 (9): 3484–3488.

Gilliland, S. E. 1990. Health and nutritional benefits from lactic acid bacteria. *FEMS Microbiol Rev* 87:175–188.

Gilliland, S. E., and D. K. Walker. 1989. Factors to consider when selecting a culture of *Lactobacillus acidophilus* as a dietary adjunct to produce a hypocholesteremic effect in humans. *J Dairy Sci* 73:905–911.

Gilliland, S. E., C. R. Nelson, and C. Maxwell. 1985. Assimilation of cholesterol by *Lactobacillus acidophilus*. *Appl Environ Microbiol* 49:377–381.

Gilliland, S. E., and H. S. Kim. 1984. Effect of viable starter culture bacteria in yogurt on lactose utilization in humans. *J Dairy Sci* 67:1–6.

Gilliland, Stanley E. 2012. *Technological & commercial applications of lactic acid bacteria: Health & nutritional benefits in dairy products*. Oklahoma State University, USA. ftp://ftp.fao.org/es/esn/food/Gilli.pdf.

Goyal, N., and D. N. Gandhi. 2008. Whey, a carrier of probiotics against diarrhoea. www.dairyscience.info/index.php/probiotics/110-whey-probiotics.html.

Liang, J., B. Z. Han, et al. 2008. Effects of soaking, germination and fermentation on phytic acid, total and in vitro soluble zinc in brown rice. *Food Chemistry* 110:821–828.

Nagel, R. 2010. Living with phytic acid. Preparing grains, nuts, seeds, and beans for maximum nutrition. *Wise Traditions in Food, Farming and the Healing Arts* 11(1). http://www.westonaprice.org/food-features/living-with-phytic-acid.

Parvez, S., K. A. Malik, et al. 2006. Probiotics and their fermented food products are beneficial for health. *Journal of Applied Microbiology* 100 (6): 1171–85.

Suma, H. 2002. Prevent heart attack and stroke with potent enzyme that dissolves deadly blood clots in hours. *Health Sciences Institute* (March) 1:83–93.

Wilder, B. Grains, nuts, seeds & legumes must be properly prepared. www.healingnaturallybybee.com/articles/foods18.php.

Wong, J. M., R. de Souza, et al. 2006. Colonic health: Fermentation and short chain fatty acids. *J Clin Gastroenterol* 40 (3): 235–243.

CHAPTER 5

Campbell-McBride, N. 2010. *Gut and psychology syndrome: Natural treatment for autism, dyspraxia, A.D.D., dyslexia, A.D.H.D., depression, schizophrenia*. Cambridge, UK: Medinform Publishing.

Drouault, S., and G. Corthier. 2001. Health effects of lactic acid bacteria ingested in fermented milk. *Vet Res* 32 (2): 101–117.

Gilliland, S. E. 1990. Health and nutritional benefits from lactic acid bacteria. *FEMS Microbial Rev* 87:175–188.

Gilliland, S. E., and H. S. Kim. 1984. Effect of viable starter culture bacteria in yogurt on lactose utilization in humans. *J Dairy Sci* 67:1–6.

Kathein, J. 2012. *Old World fermented foods vital to healthy living and nutritional healing*. Béland Organic Foods. Retrieved from http://belandorganicfoods.com/bof/organic-products/kartheins-organic-sauerkraut/fermented-foods.

Kemperman, R. A., et al. 2010. Novel approaches for analysing gut microbes and dietary polyphenols: Challenges and opportunities. *Microbiology* (November) 156 (Pt 11): 3224–3231.

Lawrence, R. 2007. *Fermentation and its health benefits*. Retrieved from www.transformyourhealth.com/webnewsletters/oct07/fermentationhealthbenefitsarticle.htm.

Manach, C., et al. 2004. Polyphenols: Food sources and bioavailability. *AJCN* 79 (5): 727–747.

Peñas E., et al. 2010. Chemical evaluation and sensory quality of sauerkrauts obtained by natural and induced fermentations at different NaCl levels from *Brassica oleracea* Var. *capitata* Cv. *Bronco* grown in eastern Spain. Effect of storage. *J Agric Food Chem* 58 (6): 3549–3557.

Perez-Jimenez, J., et al. 2010. Identification of the 100 richest dietary sources of polyphenols: An application of the Phenol-Explorer database. *Eur J Clin Nutr* 64 (S3): S112–S120.

Rechner, A. R., et al. 2004. Colonic metabolism of dietary polyphenols: Influence of structure on microbial fermentation products. Free radical. *Biology and Medicine* 36 (2): 212–225.

Ripudaman, S. Beniwal, et al. 2003. A randomized trial of yogurt for prevention of antibiotic-associated diarrhea. *Digestive Diseases and Sciences* 48 (10): 2077–2082.

Shurtleff W., A. Aoyagi. 1976. *The book of miso*. Kanagawa, Japan: Autumn Press.

Steinkraus, K. H. 1996. *Handbook of indigenous fermented foods*, 2nd ed. New York: Marcel Dekker.

Wang, H. L., D. I. Ruttle, and C. W. Hesseltine. 1969. Antibiotic compound from a soybean product fermented by *Rhizopus oligosporus*. *Proc Soc Exp Biol Med* 131:579–583.

Wigmore, Ann. www.annwigmore.org/index.html.

CHAPTER 6

Eisenstein, C. 2003. Old-fashioned, healthy, lacto-fermented soft drinks: The real thing. *Wise Traditions in Food, Farming and the Healing Arts* (Spring).

Fallon, S., and M. G. Enig. 2001. *Nourishing traditions: The cookbook that challenges politically correct nutrition and the diet dictocrats*, 2nd ed. Washington, DC: NewTrends Publishing.

Harmon, W. 2012. *Complete idiot's guide to fermenting foods*. New York: Alpha Books.

Hobbs, C. 1995. *Kombucha: The essential guide*. Santa Cruz, CA: Botanica Press.

Katz, S. E. 2003. *Wild fermentation: The flavor, nutrition, and craft of live-culture foods*. White River Junction, VT: Chelsea Green.

Kaufmann, K. 1995. *Kombucha rediscovered: A guide to the medicinal benefits of an ancient healing tea*. BC, Canada: Alive Books.

------. 2005. *Making sauerkraut and pickled vegetables at home*. Summertown, TN: Alive Books.

Leader, D. 2007. *Local breads: Sourdough and whole-grain recipes from Europe's best artisan bakers*. New York: W. W. Norton.

Man-Jo, K., et al. 1999. *The kimchi cookbook: Fiery flavors and cultural history of Korea's national dish*. North Clarendon, VT: Periplus.

Marianski, S., and A. Marianski. 2008. *The art of making fermented sausages*. Denver, CO: Outskirts Press.

Pitchford, P. 2002. *Healing with whole foods*, 3rd ed. Berkeley, CA: North Atlantic Books.

Saxelby, C., Foodwatch Nutrition Center. 2002. Top 100 foods for polyphenols (June). www.foodwatch.com.au.

Shephard, S. 2001. *Pickled, potted, and canned*. New York: Simon & Schuster.

Shurtleff, W., and A. Aoyagi. 1976. *The book of miso*. Kanagawa, Japan: Autumn Press.

------. 1979. *The book of tempeh*. New York: Harper & Row.

------. 2007. *History of soybeans and soyfoods: 1100 BC to the 1980s*. Lafayette, CA: Soyinfo Center.

Glossary

acidic: Having a pH of less than 7.

acidification: The process of producing acidity. Frequently the result of fermentation and part of how fermentation safely preserves food.

aerobic bacteria: Bacteria that require oxygen.

alkaline: Basic; having a pH of more than 7.

amino acids: The building blocks of proteins. Amino acids band together in chains to form a vast variety of proteins. A total of twenty different kinds of amino acids form proteins. Nine of these twenty are called "essential" for humans because they cannot be made by the human body and must be taken in as food.

anaerobic: The absence of oxygen or the absence of a need for oxygen.

anemia: The condition of having fewer than the normal number of red blood cells or hemoglobin in the blood, resulting in diminished oxygen transport. Anemia has many causes, including deficiencies of iron, vitamin B12, or folate; bleeding; abnormal hemoglobin formation (e.g., sickle cell anemia); rupture of red blood cells (hemolytic anemia); and bone marrow diseases.

antibiotic: Antibacterial; a compound or substance that kills or slows the growth of bacteria.

antibodies: Specialized proteins produced by white blood cells (lymphocytes) that recognize and bind to foreign proteins or pathogens in order to neutralize them or mark them for destruction.

antihistamine: A chemical that blocks the effect of histamine in susceptible tissues. Histamine is released by immune cells during an allergic reaction and during infection with viruses that cause the common cold. Histamine interacts with the mucous membranes of the eyes and nose, resulting in the watery eyes and runny nose often accompanying allergies and colds. Antihistamines can help alleviate such symptoms.

antioxidant: Any substance that prevents or reduces damage caused by free radicals.

apoptosis: Gene-directed cell death or programmed cell death that occurs when age, condition, or state of cell health dictates. Cells that die by apoptosis do not usually elicit the inflammatory responses that are associated with the death of cells. Cancer cells are resistant to apoptosis.

Aspergillus: A genus of mold frequently used in the Asian traditions of fermenting grains and legumes.

autoimmune: A condition in which the body's immune system reacts against its own tissues.

backslopping: Introducing a small part of a previous batch into the new batch in any fermentation process.

bacteria: Single-celled organisms that can exist independently, symbiotically (in cooperation with another organism), or parasitically (dependent upon another organism, sometimes to the detriment of the other organism).

benign: Noncancerous

bioavailability: The degree and rate at which an administered compound reaches the systemic circulation and is transported to the site of action (target tissue).

brine: Salt water used as a medium for pickling and preservation.

butyric acid: Fatty acid occurring in the form of esters found in animal fat and some plant fats. Butyric acid is produced on a large scale by the fermentation of starch or sugar.

cancer: Abnormal cells, which have a tendency to grow uncontrollably and metastasize, or spread, to other areas of the body. Cancer can involve any tissue of the body and can have different forms in one tissue. Cancer is a group of more than one hundred different diseases.

carbohydrate: Chemically, carbohydrates are neutral compounds composed of carbon, hydrogen, and oxygen. Carbohydrates come in simple forms known as sugars and complex forms, such as starches and fiber. Considered a macronutrient because carbohydrates provide a significant source of calories (energy) in the diet.

carcinogen: A cancer-causing agent.

cardiovascular: Referring to the heart and blood vessels.

cataract: Clouding of the lens of the eye that can impair vision.

celiac disease: Also known as celiac sprue, celiac disease is an inherited disease in which the intestinal lining is inflamed in response to the ingestion of the protein gluten. Treatment of celiac disease involves the avoidance of gluten, which is present in many grains, including wheat, rye, barley, and sometimes oats. Inflammation and atrophy of the lining of the small intestine leads to impaired nutrient absorption.

cholesterol: A compound that is an integral structural component of cell membranes and a precursor in the synthesis of steroid hormones. Dietary cholesterol is obtained from animal sources, but cholesterol is also synthesized by the liver. Cholesterol is carried in the blood.

chronic fatigue syndrome: A condition of severe, continued tiredness that is not relieved by rest and is not directly caused by other medical conditions.

collagen: A fibrous protein that is the basis for the structure of skin, tendon, bone, cartilage, and all other connective tissue.

colon: The portion of the large intestine that extends from the end of the small intestine to the rectum. The colon removes water from digested food after it has passed through the small intestine and stores the remaining stool until it can be evacuated.

Crohn's disease: An inflammatory bowel disease that usually affects the lower part of the small intestine or upper part of the colon but may affect any part of the gastrointestinal tract.

culture: See *starter culture*.

curing: Various food preservation and flavoring processes, especially of meat or fish, performed by adding a combination of salt, nitrates, nitrite, or sugar. Many curing processes involve smoking, flavoring, or cooking. The use of food dehydration was the earliest form of food curing.

cytokines: Small cell-signaling protein molecules that are secreted by numerous cells and are a category of signaling molecules used extensively in intercellular communication.

douchi: A traditional salt-fermented food made of soy; popular in China.

dysbiosis: An imbalance of intestinal bacteria. The word "dysbiosis" was first popularized by Dr. Eli Metchnikoff, who theorized that all disease begins in the digestive tract because of an imbalance of intestinal bacteria. It came from the opposite term, *symbiosis*, meaning "living together in mutual harmony," and *dys*, meaning "not."

endotoxin: Toxins released by certain bacteria.

enzyme: A biological catalyst; that is, a substance that increases the speed of a chemical reaction without being changed in the overall process. Enzymes are vitally important to the regulation of the chemistry of cells and organisms.

essential fatty acids (EFAs): Fatty acids that humans and other animals must ingest because the body requires them for good health but cannot make them on its own.

fatty acids: An organic acid molecule consisting of a chain of carbon molecules and a carboxylic acid (COOH) group. Fatty acids are found in fat, oil, and as components of a number of essential lipids, such as phospholipids and triglycerides. Fatty acids can be burned by the body for energy.

fermentation: An anaerobic process that involves the breakdown of dietary components to yield energy.

fibromyalgia (FM or FMS): A medical disorder characterized by chronic widespread pain and allodynia, a heightened and painful response to pressure.

fructooligosaccharide (FOS): A type of fiber that acts as a prebiotic in your intestines to feed the beneficial microflora.

free radical: A very reactive atom or molecule typically possessing a single unpaired electron.

gastrointestinal: Referring to or affecting the digestive tract, which includes the mouth, pharynx (throat), esophagus, stomach, and intestines.

gluten: A protein found in many grains, including wheat, rye, barley, spelt, faro, triticale, and kamut. Oats processed in the same manufacturing plant as gluten grains can sometimes be contaminated by gluten.

gout: A condition characterized by abnormally high blood levels of uric acid (urate). Urate crystals may form in joints, resulting in inflammation and pain. They may also form in the kidneys and urinary tract, resulting in kidney stones. The tendency to develop elevated blood uric acid levels and gout is often inherited.

high-density lipoprotein (HDL): A form of cholesterol that helps keep the arteries clear and the heart healthy.

hydrochloric acid (HCL): A colorless and odorless solution of hydrogen chloride and water. It is found in diluted amounts in the stomach of humans and animals as gastric acid to aid digestion, mainly of proteins.

immunoglobulins: A class of antibody found in mammals.

inflammation: A response to injury or infection, characterized by redness, heat, swelling, and pain. Physiologically, the inflammatory response involves a complex series of events, leading to the migration of white blood cells to the inflamed area.

interleukin: A protein molecule in the immune system that regulates the activities of white blood cells (leukocytes, often lymphocytes) that are responsible for immunity.

intestinal permeability: The result of damage to the lining or mucosal barrier of the digestive tract, resulting in food substances or larger molecules passing through the walls directly into the bloodstream.

inulin: A group of naturally occurring polysaccharides produced by plants. They belong to a class of dietary fibers known as fructans.

lactic acid: The acid produced by bacteria during fermentation. The most important lactic acid is *Lactobacillus*, from which it gets its name.

lacto-fermentation: A natural way of culturing, or pickling, a food. "Lacto" comes *Lactobacillus*, the natural, beneficial bacteria the method uses. *Lactobacillus* converts the carbohydrates from vegetables, fruits, grains, and other foods into lactic acid, which prevents harmful organisms from flourishing and encourages beneficial microflora to thrive.

lactose: A disaccharide sugar that is found most notably in milk and is formed from galactose and glucose.

leaky gut syndrome: A condition that affects the lining of the intestines. Also called increased intestinal permeability, it is the result of damage to the intestinal lining, making it less able to protect the internal environment or to absorb the needed nutrients.

legumes: Members of the large family of plants known as Leguminosae. In this context the term refers to the fruits or seeds of leguminous plants (e.g., peas and beans) that are used for food.

leukocytes: White blood cells. Leukocytes are part of the immune system. Monocytes, lymphocytes, neutrophils, basophils, and eosinophils are different types of leukocytes.

lipids: A chemical term for fats. Lipids found in the human body include fatty acids, phospholipids, and triglycerides.

low-density lipoprotein (LDL): LDLs transport cholesterol from the liver to the tissues of the body. Elevated serum LDL cholesterol is associated with increased cardiovascular disease risk.

lymphocytes: Leukocytes (white blood cells) that play important roles in the immune system. T lymphocytes (T cells) differentiate into cells that can kill infected cells or activate other cells in the immune system. B lymphocytes (B cells) differentiate into cells that produce antibodies.

macronutrient: Nutrients required in relatively large amounts; macronutrients include carbohydrates, proteins, and lipids.

macrophage: A type of white blood cell that begins its life as a monocyte. A monocyte is produced in the bone marrow and circulates throughout the bloodstream.

malabsorption: Difficulty digesting or absorbing nutrients from food.

malignant: Cancerous.

metabolism: The sum of the processes (reactions) by which a substance is assimilated and incorporated into the body or detoxified and excreted from the body.

micronutrient: A nutrient required by the body in small amounts, such as a vitamin or a mineral.

mineral: Nutritionally significant element. Elements are composed of only one kind of atom. Minerals are inorganic, meaning they do not contain carbon, unlike vitamins and other organic compounds.

natural killer cells (NK cells, K cells, and killer cells): A type of lymphocyte (white blood cell) and a component of the innate immune system.

neurotransmitter: A chemical that is released from a nerve cell and results in the transmission of an impulse to another nerve cell or organ (e.g., a muscle). Acetylcholine, dopamine, norepinephrine, and serotonin are neurotransmitters.

neutrophils: White blood cells that internalize and destroy pathogens, such as bacteria.

optimum health: Freedom from disease, as well as the ability of an individual to function physically and mentally at his or her best.

organic: Food produced without the use of pesticides or antibiotics.

oxidative stress: A condition in which the effects of pro-oxidants (e.g. free radicals, reactive oxygen and reactive nitrogen species) exceed the ability of antioxidant systems to neutralize them.

pasteurization: A process of heating a food, usually liquid, to a specific temperature for a predefined length of time and then immediately cooling it.

pathogen: Disease-causing agents, such as viruses or bacteria.

peptides: The building blocks of protein, peptides are small structures built by amino acids.

pH: A measure of acidity or alkalinity.

phagocyte: A specialized cell, such as a macrophage, that engulfs and digests invading microorganisms through the process of phagocytosis.

pickling: Also known as brining, this is the process of preserving food by anaerobic fermentation in a brine to produce lactic acid.

polyphenols: Antioxidants found in fruits, vegetables, legumes, and seeds that assist in addressing and reversing the damage caused by oxidative stress.

prebiotics: Nondigestible food ingredients that stimulate growth and activity of bacteria in the digestive system in ways that are beneficial to health.

probiotic: Live microorganisms that, when administered in sufficient amounts, benefit the overall health of the host.

protein: A complex organic molecule composed of amino acids in a specific order. The order is determined by the sequence of nucleic acids in a gene coding for the protein. Proteins are required for the structure, function, and regulation of the body's cells, tissues, and organs, and each protein has unique functions.

schizophrenia: A debilitating brain disorder that affects about 1 percent of the world's population. Symptoms may include hallucinations, delusions, thought disorders, disorders of movement, cognitive deficits, flat affect, lack of pleasure, or impaired ability to speak, plan, or interact with others. Although its cause is not known, schizophrenia is thought to result from a combination of genetic and environmental factors.

SCOBY: An acronym for symbiotic culture of bacteria and yeast that's used to make probiotic beverages such as kombucha.

scurvy: A disorder caused by a lack of vitamin C. Symptoms include anemia, bleeding gums, tooth loss, joint pain, and fatigue. Scurvy is treated by supplying foods high in vitamin C as well as with vitamin C supplements.

small intestine: The part of the digestive tract that extends from the stomach to the large intestine. The small intestine includes the duodenum (closest to the stomach), the jejunum, and the ileum (closest to the large intestine).

starter culture: A preparation to assist the beginning of the fermentation process for various foods and fermented drinks. It refers to microbiological starters that actually perform fermentation. These starters generally consist of a cultivation medium—such as grains, seeds, or nutrient liquids—that has been well colonized by the microorganisms being used for fermentation.

supplement: A nutrient or phytochemical supplied in addition to what is obtained in the diet.

triglycerides: Lipids consisting of three fatty acid molecules bound to a glycerol backbone. Triglycerides are the principal form of fat in the diet, although they are also synthesized endogenously (within the body). Triglycerides are stored in fat and tissue, and are the principal storage form of fat. Elevated serum triglycerides are a risk factor for cardiovascular disease.

villi: The fingerlike protrusions in the small intestine that help absorb nutrients more efficiently. People with celiac disease have fewer or deficient villi, meaning they are unable to absorb all the nutrients they need.

virus: A microorganism that cannot grow or reproduce apart from a living cell. Viruses invade living cells and use the synthetic processes of infected cells to survive and replicate.

vitamin: An organic (carbon-containing) compound necessary for normal physiological function that cannot be synthesized in adequate amounts and must therefore be obtained in the diet.

yeast: A broad group of fungi that metabolize sugars into alcohol.

Recommended Books

Campbell-McBride, Natasha. *Gut and Psychology Syndrome: Natural Treatment for Autism, Dyspraxia, A.D.D., Dyslexia, A.D.H.D., Depression, Schizophrenia*. Cambridge, UK: Medinform Publishing, 2010.

Fallon, Sally, and Mary G. Enig. *Nourishing Traditions: The Cookbook That Challenges Politically Correct Nutrition and the Diet Dictocrats*. 2nd ed. Washington, DC: NewTrends Publishing, 2001.

Harmon, Wardeh. *The Complete Idiot's Guide to Fermenting Foods*. New York: Alpha Books, 2007.

Huffnagle, Gary B. with Sarah Wernick. *The Probiotics Revolution: The Definitive Guide to Safe, Natural Health Solutions Using Probiotic and Prebiotic Foods and Supplements*. New York: Bantam Books, 2007.

Katz, Sandor Ellix. *Wild Fermentation: The Flavor, Nutrition, and Craft of Live-Culture Foods*. White River Junction, VT: Chelsea Green Publishing, 2003.

Lewin, Alex. *Real Food Fermentation: Preserving Whole Fresh Food with Live Cultures in Your Home Kitchen*. Beverly, MA: Quarry Books, 2012.

Pitchford, Paul. *Healing with Whole Foods: Asian Traditions and Modern Nutrition*. Berkeley, CA: North Atlantic Books, 2003.

Schmid, Ronald F. *The Untold Story of Milk: The History, Politics and Science of Nature's Perfect Food: Raw Milk from Pasture-Fed Cows*. Washington, DC: NewTrends Publishing, 2009.

Resources

STARTER CULTURES

Cultures for Health
www.culturesforhealth.com
Nondairy starter cultures, water kefir grains, dairy kefir grains, kombucha SCOBYs, soy cultures, sourdough starters, gluten-free sourdough starters. Also carries Natto Spores (aka Natto-Moto) for the starter cultures used with soybeans to make traditional Japanese natto fresh at home.

Kombucha Kamp
http://store.kombuchakamp.com/Kombucha-Culture-SCOBY.html
Large, fresh kombucha cultures (never dehydrated) packed in strong starter tea, with free shipping and full support from "the Kombucha Mamma" included. Guaranteed to brew inexpensive, healthful, delicious homemade kombucha in 7 days.

Royal Kombucha
www.royalkombucha.com
Kombucha starter kits

Wilderness Family Naturals
www.wildernessfamilynaturals.com/category/culturing-products.php
Make your own yogurt, kefir, and fermented vegetables with these culture starters. Also carries rennet for cheese making and electric yogurt makers.

Wise Choice Market
www.wisechoicemarket.com
Caldwell's unique starter culture for vegetables will help you make your own delicious raw cultured vegetables at home.

WILD AND SUSTAINABLY FARMED SEAFOOD

Monterey Bay Aquarium
www.montereybayaquarium.org/cr/seafoodwatch.aspx
Provides information on which seafood has the fewest contaminants and least mercury content.

BEST CHOICES FOR PRODUCE

Environmental Working Group
www.ewg.org/foodnews
Learn which produce are the most chemically laden.

MONOSODIUM GLUTAMATE (MSG)

Holistic Medicine—Toxicity Web Page
www.holisticmed.com/msg
Learn which foods contain MSG.

Truth in Labeling
www.truthinlabeling.org/hiddensources.html
Learn which foods have MSG hidden in them.

NUTRITION EDUCATION

Weston A. Price Foundation
www.westonaprice.org
Information on wise traditions in food, farming, and the healing arts.

About the Author

Deirdre Rawlings, Ph.D., N.D., M.H., C.N.C., is a board-certified traditional Naturopathic Doctor (AANM), Certified Nutrition Counselor, Certified Sports Nutritionist, Master Herbalist, and Certified Health Coach. Through her two websites, http://FoodsforFibromyalgia.com and http://Nutri-Living.com, she offers wellness education, healthy cooking programs, health retreats, and health coaching on subjects ranging from longevity and hormone balance to disease prevention, weight loss, and stress management.

Dr. Rawlings has written hundreds of health and nutrition articles and published four books that cover topics such as fibromyalgia, hypertension, sugar addiction, and digestive health. Through her writings, she shares the latest scientific health principles and practices to help people experience the healing powers of food and nutrition.

Acknowledgments

I'd like to thank the utterly brilliant scientists and fermentationists whose work and writings on the subject of microbiology and bacteria paved the way for this book. Without them, this book could not have been written, or at least would not have contained as vast a discussion on an "old" topic that is continually evolving and being made "new": Gary Hufnagle, Ph.D., Sarkis Mazmanian, Ph.D., Elie Metchnikov, Ph.D., to name only a few.

To Jill Alexander, senior editor at Fair Winds Press and the person who first proposed the concept of this book; and to my editors and designers who turned this work into a union of cohesion: Heather Godin, Kathie Alexander, John Gettings, Jennifer Kushnier, Andrea Rud, and Karen Levy.

To my family and friends who supported me and were kind and understanding toward me throughout the project: Jonathan, Jeanne, Ben, Harry, Felix, and Tiger—I love you. And to my beloved stepfather, Joe, who first instilled in me my love of fermented foods, and educated me on their benefits all those years ago—thank you and God bless.

Index